Based on 2 of the world's greatest traditional medical care systems

BORDERLESS DOCTOR

Dr. Biswaroop Roy Chowdhury

Dr. Giang Phung Tuan

DIAMOND BOOKS

Editing :
Rachna Sharma

Proofreading :
Anupama Sharma

Graphics Designer :
Shankar Singh Koranga

Cartoons :
Bijan Samaddar, Komal Singh

Edition : September 2015

Published By :
Diamond Pocket Books
X-30, Okhla Industrial Area
Tel: 011-40712100
E-mail:sales@pdp.in website: www.diamondbook.in

Design Studio:
India Book of Records
B-121, 2nd Floor, Greenfields, Faridabad-121010
Ph. 0129-2510534, 9312286540
Website : www.biswaroop.com
Email : biswaroop@biswaroop.com

Facebook:
www.facebook.com/heartmafia.official
Twitter:
https://twitter.com/biswaroopproy
Linkedin:
www.linkedin.com/pub/dr-biswaroop-roy-chowdhury/58/618/866
YouTube channel:
Dr.Biswaroop Chowdhury

Printed by : Repro Knowledgecast Limited, Thane

BORDERLESS DOCTOR
Dr. Biswaroop Roy Chowdhury | Dr. Giang Phung Tuan

DEDICATION

By Dr. Biswaroop Roy Chowdhury

Dedicated to my angel daughter Ivy,
loving wife Neerja
&
caring parents.

By Dr. Giang Phung Tuan

Dedicated to my family
who have selflessly worked hard to preserve
and propagate Vietnam's Ancient Medical wisdom
for the benefit of humanity.

From the Authors

"Being healthy is not just your right...
... it's your responsibility as well.

In this world, humans are the only animals who suffer the most part of their lifetime. Rest of the inhabitants of the planet live healthy and even die healthy. Have you ever heard a cat dying of a heart attack or a cow suffering from diabetes? And even if they get sick, their natural instincts guide them to be healthy again. For instance when a tiger gets ill, it starts consuming some specific kind of leaves.

This book is written with the intention of reclaiming your freedom from 3D's i.e. Drugs, Diseases and Doctors as well.

This book, in a step by step manner, will guide you to recover from illness and be healthy again without the intervention of modern doctors.

Dr. Gang Phung Tuan — Dr. Biswaroop Roy Chowdhury

CONTENT

SECTION -I

HOW TO EXAMINE A SICK PERSON & IDENTIFY HIS ILLNESS

SECTION -II

FIRST AID & WATER HEALING METHOD

SECTION -III
SOME VERY COMMON SICKNESSES

SECTION -IV

SOME VERY COMMON SICKNESSES

SECTION -V

SPECIAL SECTION

SECTION I

You will be able to care for the sick person, only when you are able to identify his illness. This section will teach you the methods to examine a sick person and identify his illness.

HOW TO EXAMINE A SICK PERSON & IDENTIFY HIS ILLNESS

To examine a sick person, you may follow the below mentioned protocol:

Questions

⇩

General Condition of health

⇩

Temperature

⇩

How to use a Thermometer

⇩

Various Types of Illnesses that cause

⇩

fever

⇩

Breathing (Respiration)

⇩

Pulse (Heartbeat)

⇩

Eyes

⇩

Ears

⇩

Skin

⇩

The Belly (Abdomen)

QUESTIONS

You may start asking questions to the sick person in the given order:

Q. 1 What bothers you most right now?
Q. 2 What makes you feel better or worse?
Q. 3 How and when did your sickness begin?
Q. 4 Have you had this same trouble before?
Q. 5 Has anyone else in your family or neighborhood had it?

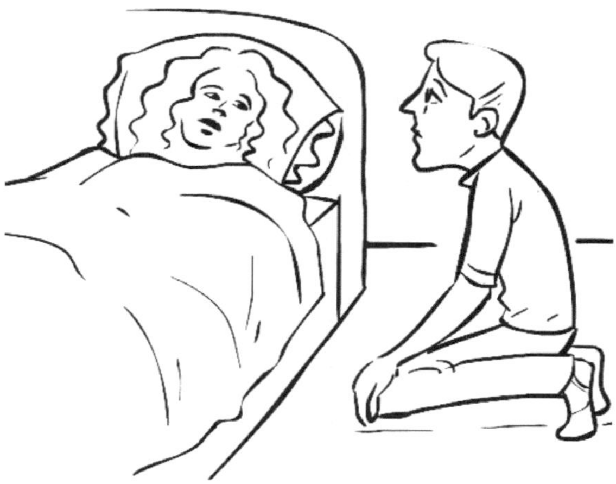

If the sick person has a pain you may ask:

Q. 1 Where does it hurt?
Q. 2 Does it hurt all the time or off and on?
Q. 3 Is the pain sharp, dull or burning?
Q. 4 Can you sleep with the pain?

GENERAL CONDITION OF HEALTH

Observe the following signs in sick person:

- How ill or weak he looks?
- How he breathes and how clear his mind seems to be?
- Does the person looks well nourished or poorly nourished?
- Has he been losing weight?
- Has anyone else in his family or neighborhood had it?

Notice the color of the eyes and skin

- Paleness; especially of the lips and inside the eyelids → Anemia.
- Darkening of skin → Starvation.
- Bluish skin; especially blueness or darkness or darkness of lips and fingernails → Breathing problems.
- Blue - gray color in an unconscious child → Cerebral Malaria.
- A gray white coloring, with cool moist skin → Shock.
- Yellow color of the skin and eyes → Jaundice.
- Lighter skin → Tuberculosis.

TEMPERATURE

Take sick person's temperature, even if he does not seem to have fever. If you do not have thermometer then:

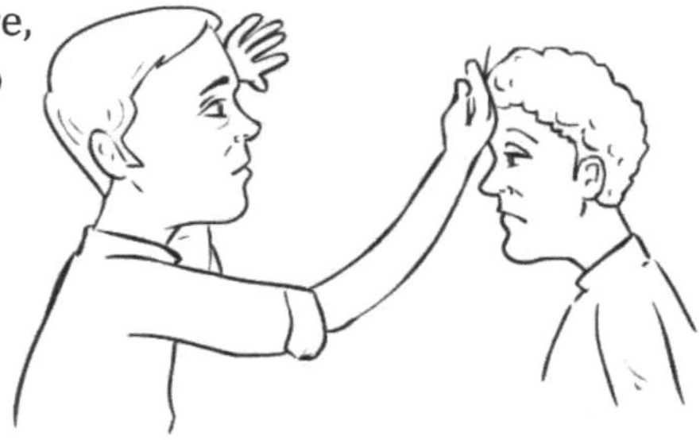

- Get an idea of the temperature by putting the back of one hand on the sick person's forehead and other on your own or that of another healthy person.

HOW TO USE A THERMOMETER:

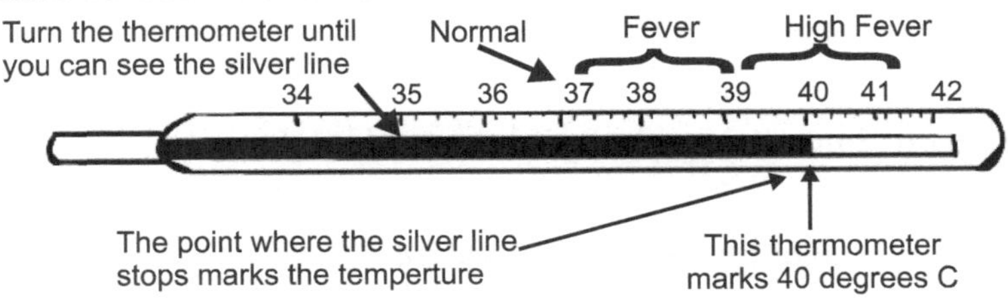

How to take the temperature:

1. Clean the thermometer well with water and alcohol. Shake it hard, with a snap of the wrist, until it reads less than 36 degrees.

2. Put the thermometer as shown below:

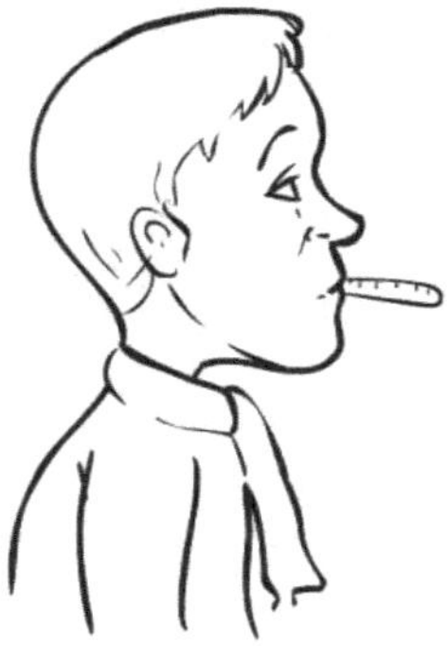

Put the thermometer under the tongue (keeping the mouth shut)

or

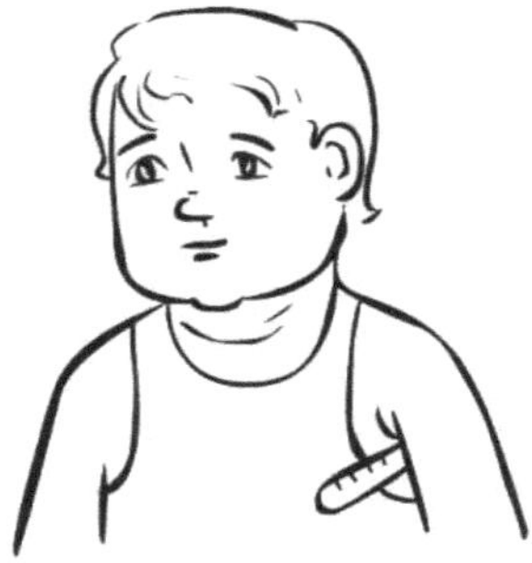

Put the thermometer in the armpit if there is danger of biting the thermometer

or

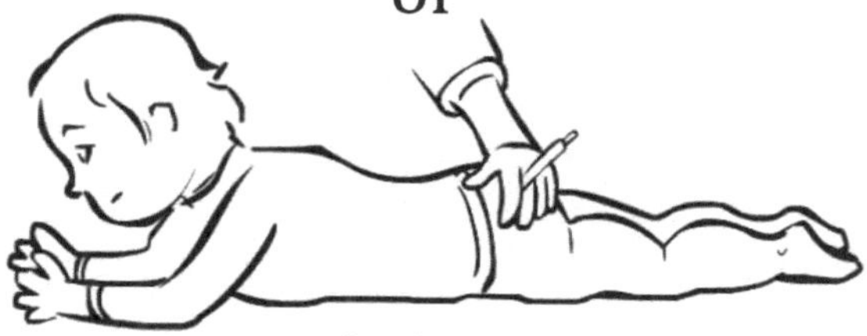

Put the thermometer carefully, in the anus of the small child (wet or grease it first)

3. Leave it there for 3 or 4 minutes.
4. Read it.
5. Wash the thermometer well with soap and water.

Variation of temperature may be because of:

- Common cold and other viral infections
- Typhoid
- Malaria
- Tuberculosis

VARIOUS TYPES OF ILLNESSES THAT CAUSES FEVER

MALARIA

Symptoms:

- Begins with weakness, chills and fever.
- Fever may come and go for a few days.

MALARIA-TYPICAL FEVER PATTERN

The solid line shows the rise and fall of temperature

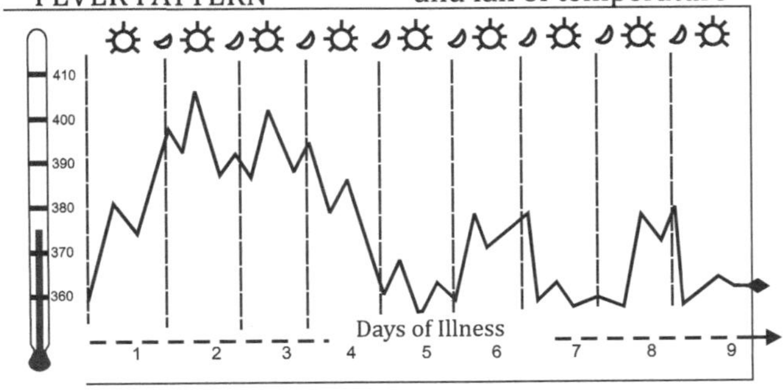

TYPHOID

Symptoms:

- Begins like a cold.
- Temperature goes up a little more each day.
- Slow pulse.
- Sometimes diarrhea and dehydration.

TYPHOID-TYPICAL FEVER PATTERN

The fever goes up a little each day.

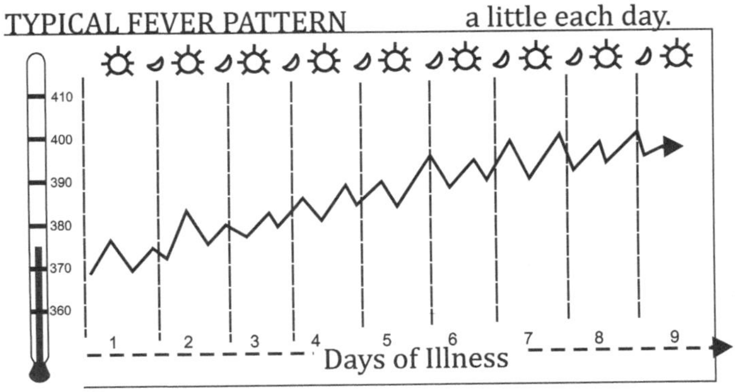

TYPHUS

Symptoms:

- Typhus begins like a bad cold.
- Rash with tiny bruises.
- The fever lasts for 2 weeks or more.

HEPATITIS

Symptoms:

- Loss of appetite.
- Nausea.
- Yellowish eyes and skin.
- Urine orange or brown and whitish stool.

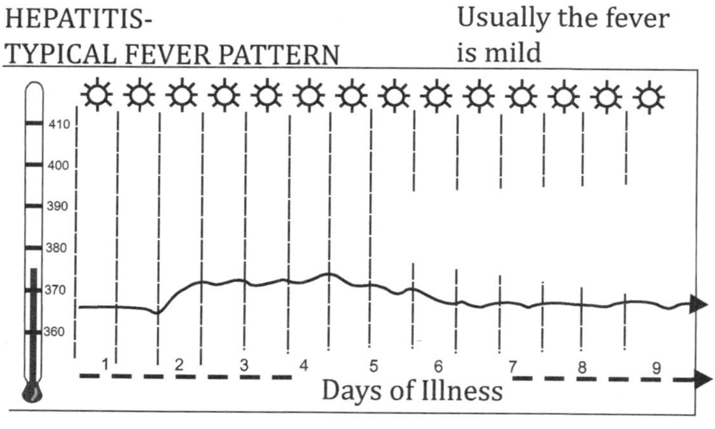

PNEUMONIA

Symptoms:

- Fast, shallow breathing.
- Temperature rises quickly.
- Cough with green, yellow or bloody mucus.

PNEUMONIA-TYPICAL FEVER PATTERN

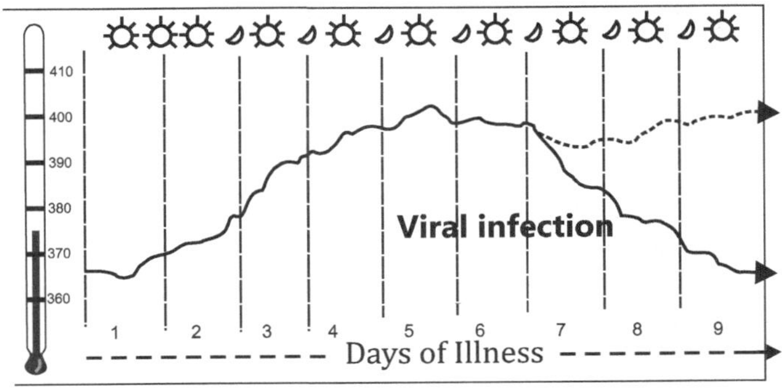

RHEUMATIC FEVER

Symptoms:

- Common in children and teenagers.
- Pain in joints.
- High fever.
- Uncontrolled movements of arms and legs.

RHEUMATIC FEVER-TYPICAL FEVER PATTERN

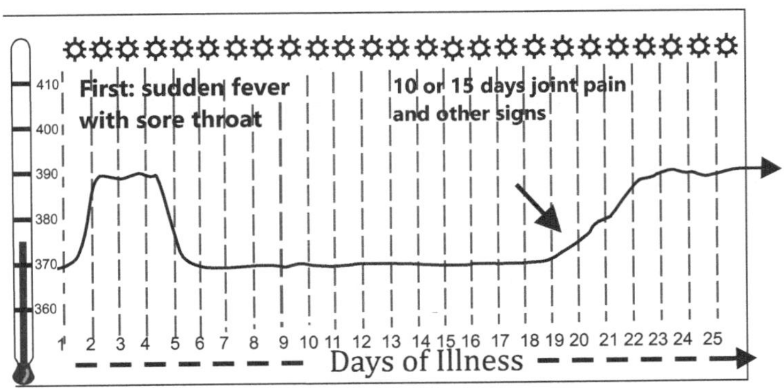

BRUCELLOSIS

Symptoms:

- Begins slowly with tiredness, headache and pain in the bones.
- Fever and sweating most common at night.

BRUCELLOSIS-
TYPICAL FEVER PATTERN

Fever comes in waves rises in the afternoon and falls at night

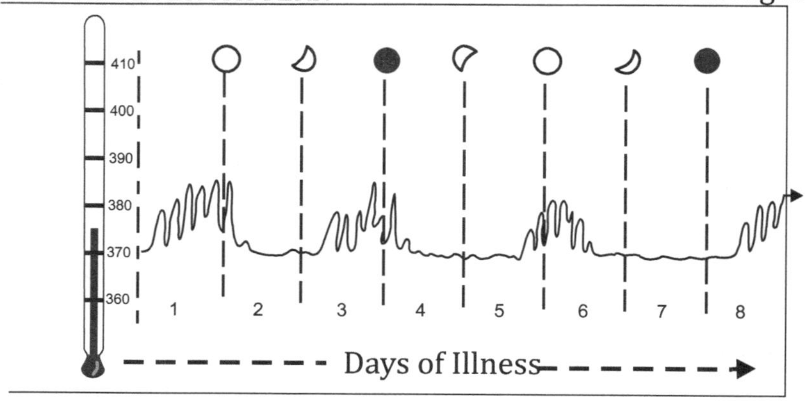

CHILDBIRTH FEVER

Symptoms:

- Begins a day or more after giving birth.
- Foul smelling vaginal discharge.

CHILD BIRTH FEVER- TYPICAL FEVER PATTERN

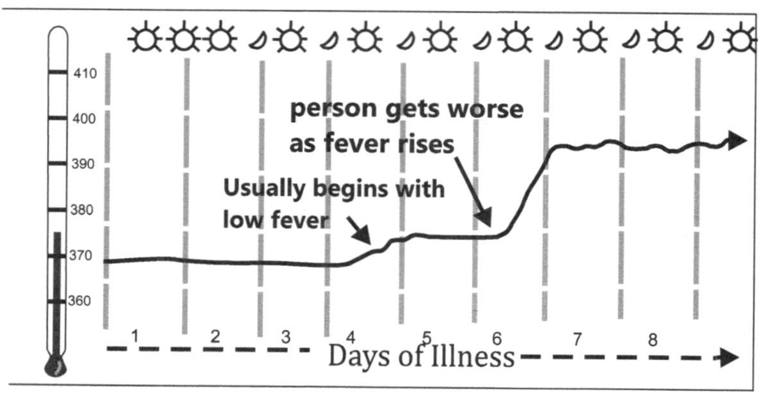

BREATHING (RESPIRATION)

Listen carefully to the sound of the breaths:

- A whistle or wheeze and difficulty in breathing out ⟶ Asthma
- A gurgling or snoring noise and difficult breathing in an unconscious person ⟶ Mucus or something else stuck in throat.

PULSE (HEARTBEAT)

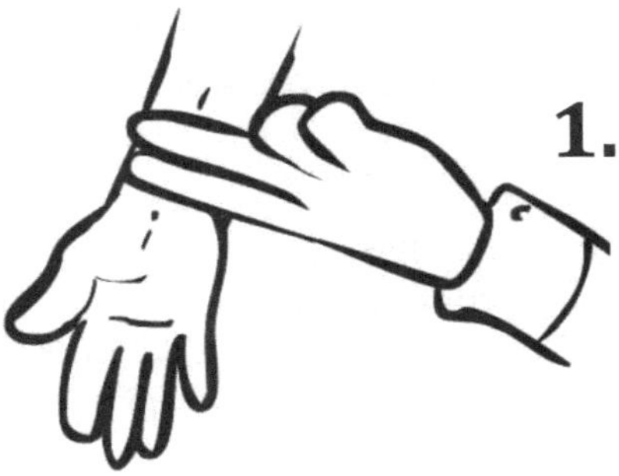

1. To take the person's pulse, put your fingers on the wrist as shown. Do not use your thumb to feel for the pulse.

2. If you cannot find the pulse in the wrist, feel for it in the neck beside the voice box.

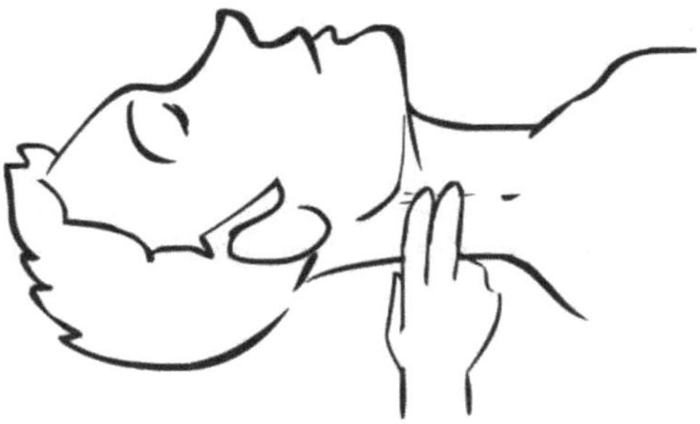

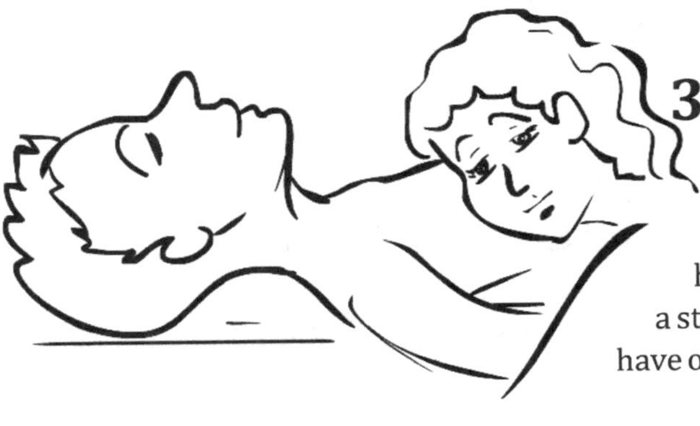

3. Or put your ear directly on the chest and listen for the heartbeat or use a stethoscope if you have one.

Normal Pulse rate for people at rest

- Adults 60 to 80 per minute
- Children 80 to 100
- Babies 100 to 140

The pulse increases 20 beats per minute for each degree rise in fever. Notice the changes in the pulse rate:

- A weak, rapid pulse → State of shock.
- A very rapid, very slow, or irregular pulse → Heart trouble.
- A relatively slow pulse in a person with high fever → Typhoid.

EYES

Look at the color of white part of the eyes. Many different problems may cause red, painful eyes as shown in the chart below:

Foreign object (bit of dirt etc. in the eye):	Usually affects one eye only, redness and pain
Burns or harmful liquids:	One or both eyes, redness and pain variable
Pink eye, Conjunctivitis: **Hay fever, trachoma, Measles:**	Usually, both eyes (may start or be worse in one) Usually reddest at outer edge Burning pain & it is usually mild
Acute glaucoma, scratch or ulcer on the cornea: Pay attention to the size and color of the pupils.	Usually one eye only, reddest next to the cornea, pain often great.

Pay attention to the size and color of the pupils.

- If they are very large → State of shock.
- If they are very large or very small → Poison or the effect of certain drugs.

- If there is white glow → Cataract or Cancer.
- If the eye with the larger pupil hurts so badly it causes vomiting → Glaucoma.
- If the eye with the smaller pupil hurts a great deal → Iritis.
- Difference in the size of the pupils of an unconscious person or a person who has had a recent head injury → Brain damage/Stroke.

EARS, THROAT AND NOSE

EARS

Symptoms:

- Redness or pus inside the ear.
- Baby cries a lot or pulls his ear often.

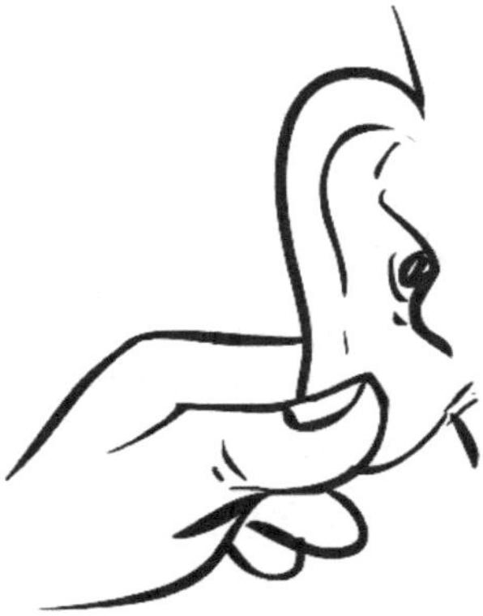

THROAT AND MOUTH:

Symptoms:

- Swelling or spots with pus.
- Redness or lumps at the back of throat.
- Inflamed gums, sore tongue.
- Rotten or abscessed teeth.

NOSE

Symptoms:

- Runny or plugged nose.
- Mucus, Pus, blood.
- Redness, swelling or bad smell.
- Sinus trouble or hay fever.

SKIN

Examine the sick person's whole body and look carefully for:

- Sores, wounds, or splinters.

- Rashes or welts.
- Spots, patches, or any unusual markings.
- Inflammation (Sign of infection with redness, heat, pain and swelling).
- Swelling or puffiness.
- Swollen lymph nodes.
- Abnormal lumps or masses.
- Unusual thinning or loss of hair or loss of its color or shine.
- Loss of eyebrows.

THE BELLY (ABDOMEN)

Observe the following signs in sick person:

- The pain is steady or whether it suddenly comes and goes.
- Is there any unusual swelling or lumps in the belly?
- Listen for gurgles in the intestines. If you hear nothing after about 2 minutes, this is a danger sign.
- Is the belly soft or hard?
- Is the pain constant with nausea?

First ask the person to point with one finger where it hurts then begin on the opposite side from the spot where he has pointed, press gently on different parts of the belly to see where it hurts most.

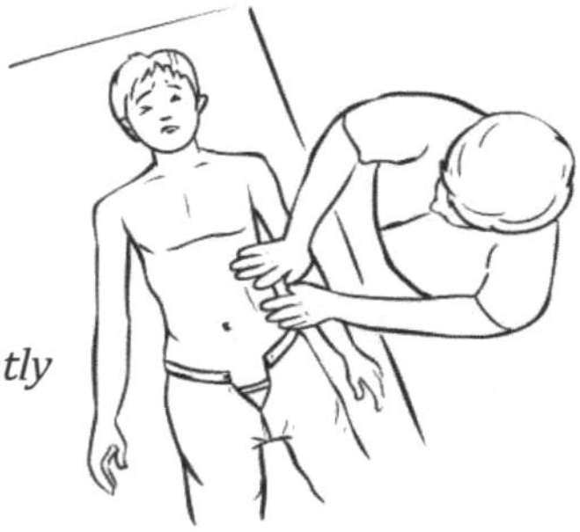

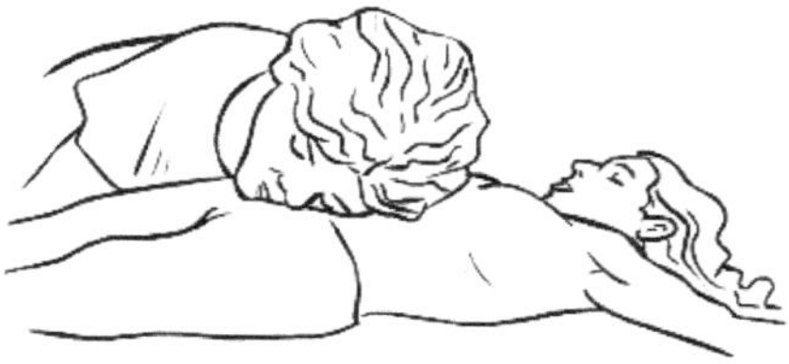

Listen for gurgles in the intestines. If you hear nothing after about 2 minutes, this is a danger sign.

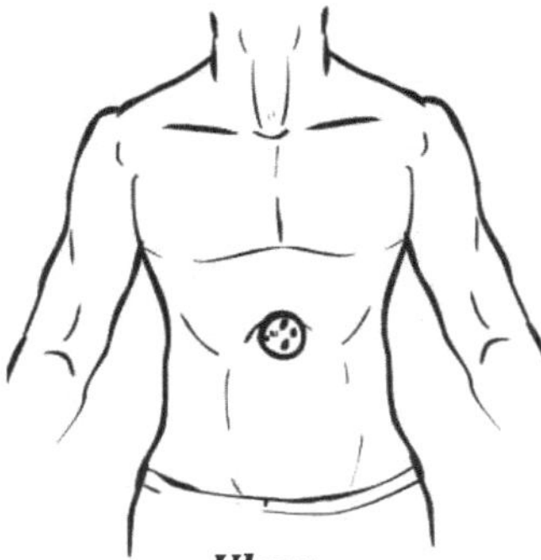

Ulcer
Pain in the pit of the stomach

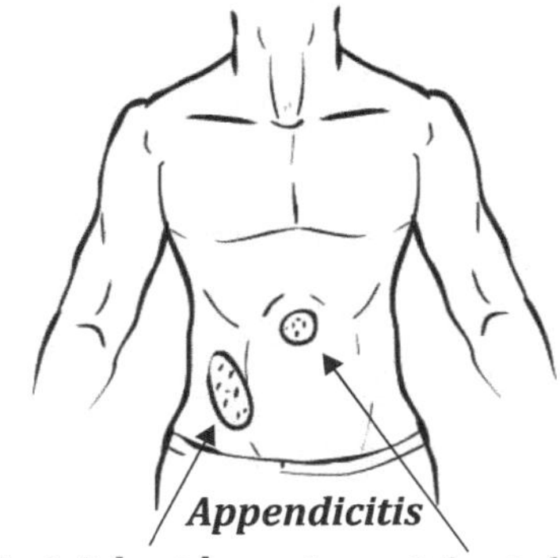

Appendicitis
First it hurt here Later it hurts here

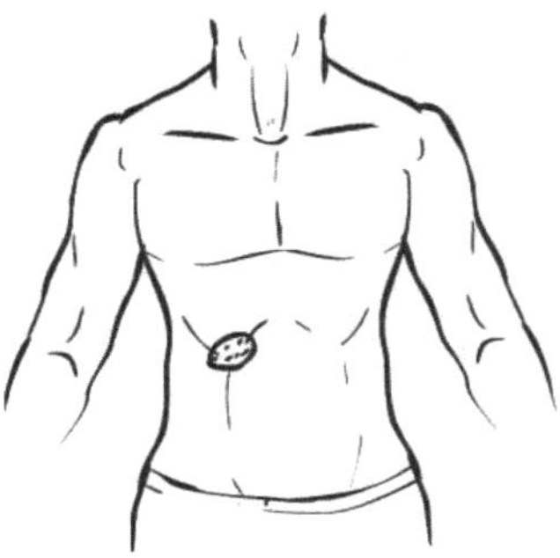

Gallbladder
Pain often reaches to the back

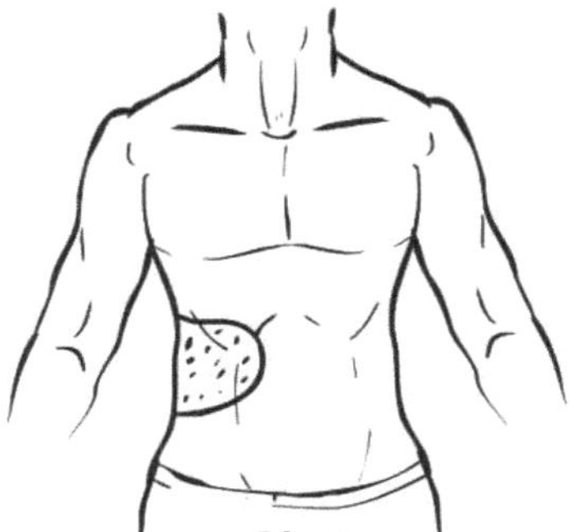

Liver
Pains here at times & it spreads to the chest

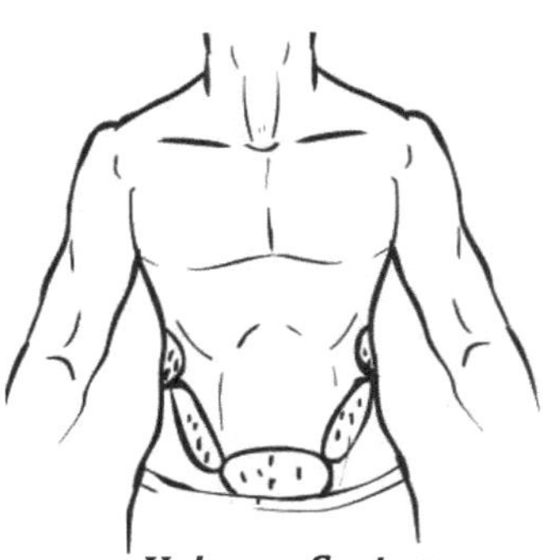

Urinary System
Mid or low back pain often goes around the waist to the lower part of the belly.

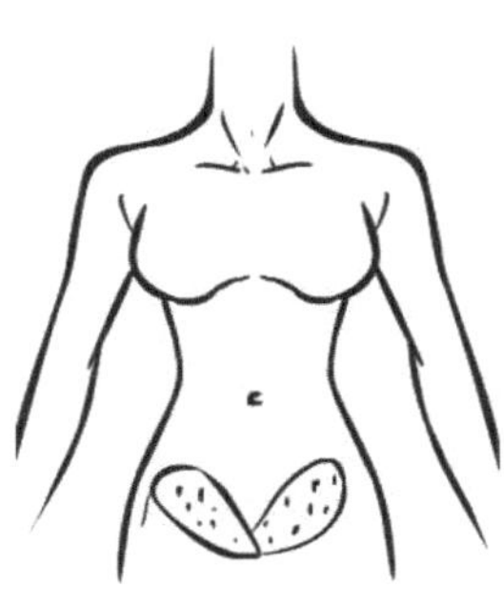

Inflammation or tumor of the ovaries
Pain on one side or both, sometimes spreading to the back

MUSCLES AND NERVES

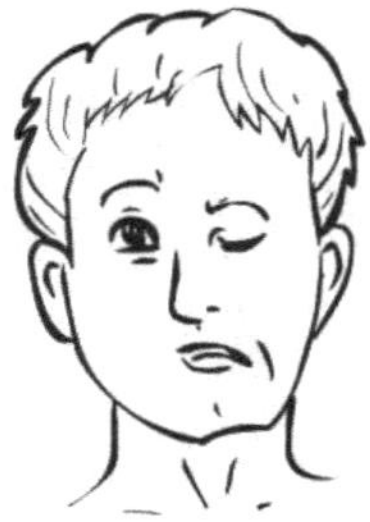

- Numbness, weakness or loss of control in part of one's body
- Drooping or weakness on one side of the face.
- Difference in thickness of arms or legs.

ARMS AND LEGS

- Look for loss of muscle.
- Notice or measure difference in the thickness of arms or legs.
- Watch how he/she walks.

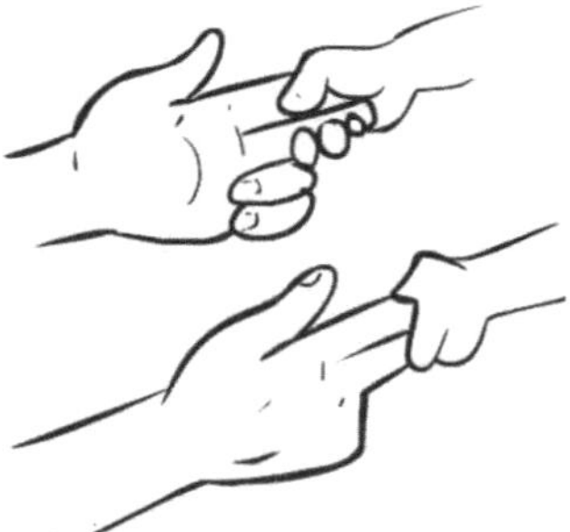

Ask him/her to squeeze your fingers to compare strength in his/her hands

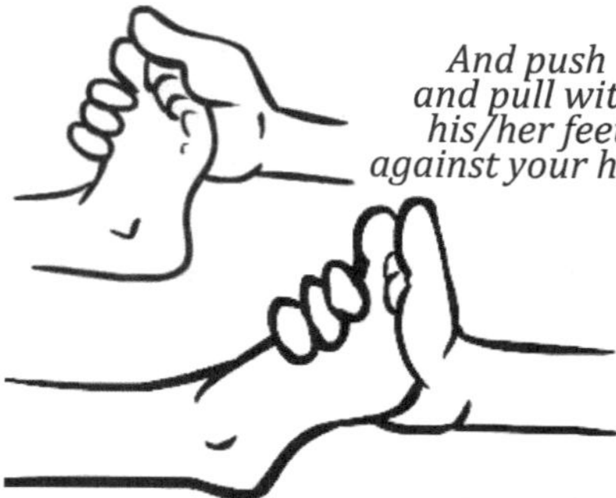

And push and pull with his/her feet against your hand

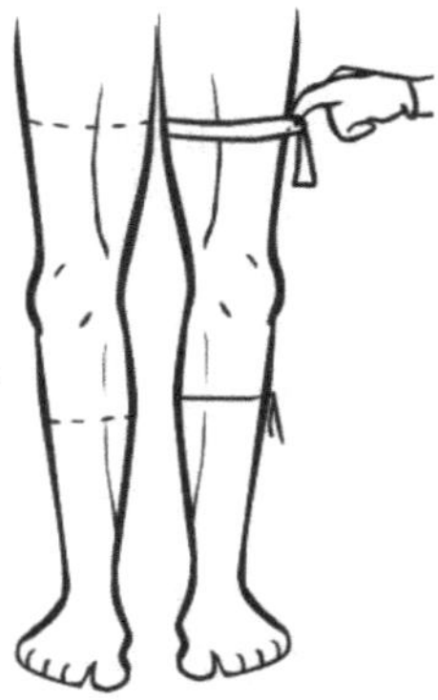

Any string or ribbon will do to check if the distance around the arms or legs is different.

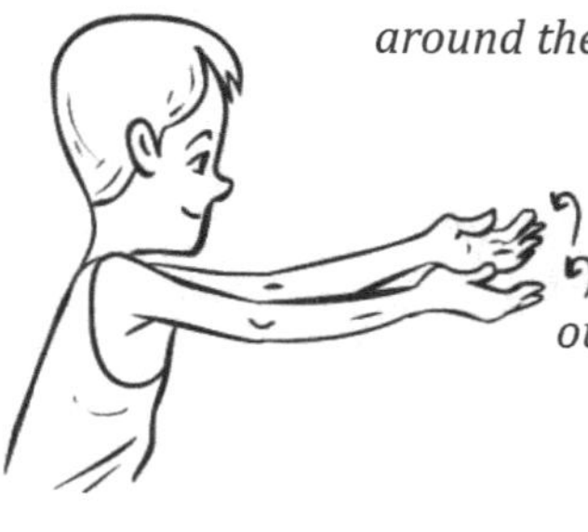

Also ask him hold his arms straight out and turn his hands up and down

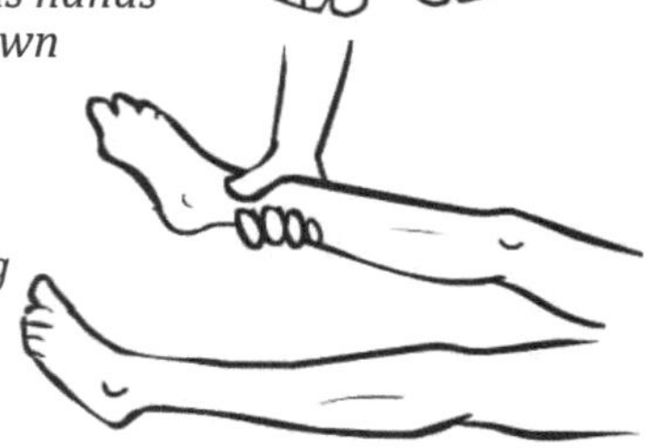

Make him lie down and lift one leg and then the other one.

Check for stiffness or tightness of different muscles

- If the jaw is stiff or it is not open → Tetanus or severe infection of throat or tooth.
- If the neck or back is stiff and bent backwards → Meningitis.
- If the child always has some stiff muscles and makes strange or jerky movements → Spastic.
- If strange or jerky movements come suddenly with the loss of consciousness → Seizures.

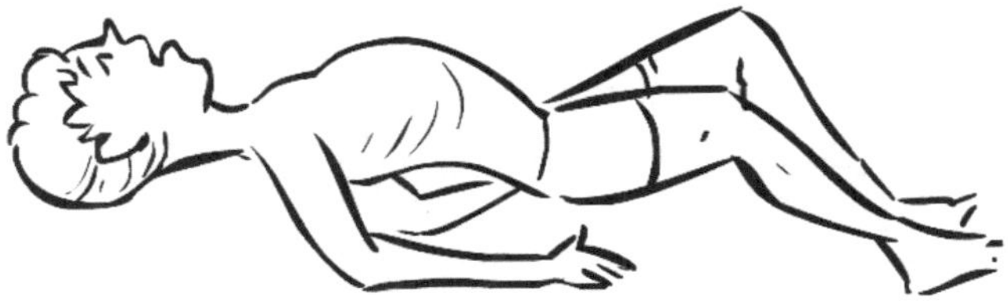

Meningitis

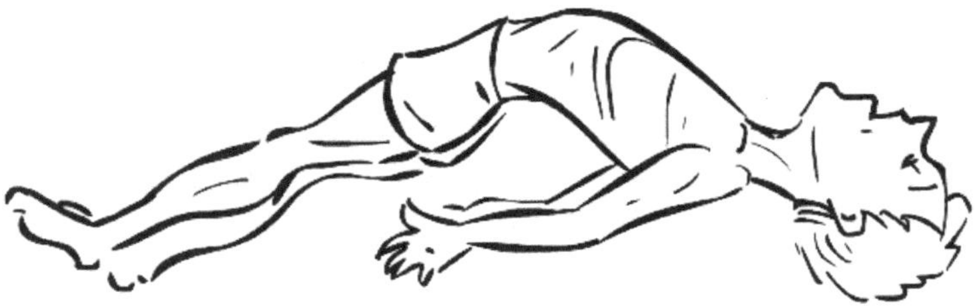

Tetanus

Check the loss of feeling in the hands, feet, or other parts of the body:

- Loss of feeling in or near spots or patches on the body → Leprosy.
- Loss of feeling in both hands and feet → Diabetes.
- Loss of feeling on one side only → Back problem.

Note:

Note:

Note:

SECTION II

This section will train you for handling the emergency situation especially when a person has hurt himself accidently. The First Aid methods given in the section will not only help you to give instant relief to the injured person but will also help you to save a life.

FIRST AID & WATER HEALING METHOD

BASIC CLEANLINESS AND PROTECTION

- Always wash hands before and after giving first aid.
- Wear gloves or a clean plastic bag on your hands to keep the blood off.
- Avoid objects soiled with blood.
- Be careful not to prick yourself with needles or other sharp objects around the person you are helping.
- Cover cuts or other wounds with dry, clean bandages to protect them.

FEVER

Recommended steps:

- Uncover him completely.
- Never wrap the child in clothing or blankets.
- Put the person in cool place & fan him.
- Give him lots of water, juices or other liquids to drink.

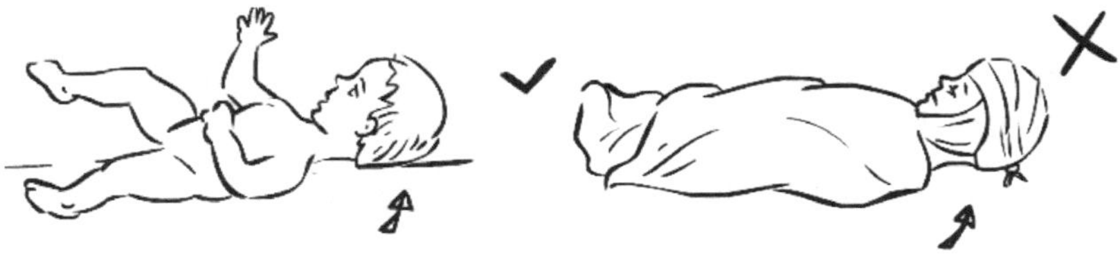

Very High Fever

Recommended steps:

- Put the person in a cool place.
- Remove all clothing.
- Fan him.
- Put cool water over him or put cloths soaked in cool water on his chest and forehead.

- Consume fruits and vegetable juice (3 times a day) alternatively every hour for a day.

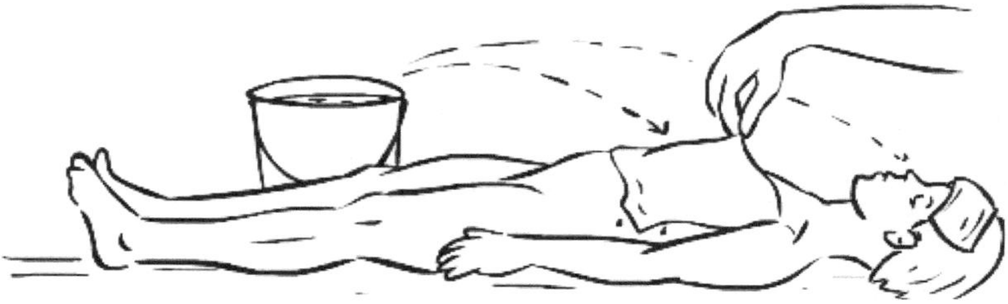

- Give him lots of water, juices or other liquids to drink.

SHOCK

Symptoms:

- Weak, rapid pulse (more than 100 per minute).
- Cold sweat, pale, cold damp skin.
- Blood pressure drops dangerously low.
- Mental confusion, weakness or loss of consciousness.

Recommended steps at the first sign of shock:

- Loosen any belts or tight clothing the person may be wearing.
- Make the person lie down with his feet a little higher than his head.
- Stop any bleeding. Use gloves or a plastic bag to keep the blood off your hands.
- If the person feels cold, cover him with blanket.
- Give him sips of water or other drinks if he is conscious and able to drink.

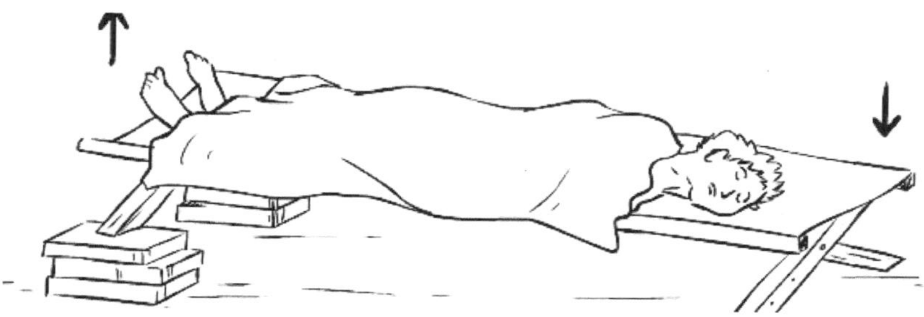

- Treat his wounds if he has any.
- Keep him calm and reassure him.

Recommended steps if the person is unconscious:

- Lay him on his side with his head low. If he seems to be choking, pull his tongue forward with your finger.
- If he has vomited, clear his mouth immediately. Be sure his head is low, tilted back to one side so that he does not breathe vomit into his lungs.
- If he has neck or spine injury, do not tilt his head or move his back.
- Do not give him anything to eat or drink until he becomes conscious.
- Handle the victim very gently.

LOSS OF CONSCIOUSNESS:

If the person is unconscious and you do not know why, immediately check each of the following:

- Is he breathing? If not, tilt his head way back and pull the jaw and tongue forward.
- Is he losing a lot of blood? If so, control the bleeding.
- Is he in shock? If so, lay him with his head lower than his feet and loosen his clothing.
- Is it a heat stroke? If so, shade him from the sun, keep his head higher than his feet and soak him with cold water and fan him.
- Never give anything by mouth to a person who is unconscious.

How to position an unconscious person:

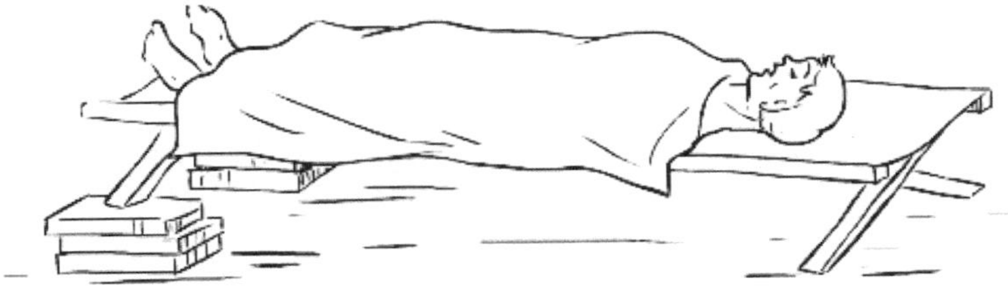

Very pale skin
(Shock, Fainting, etc.)

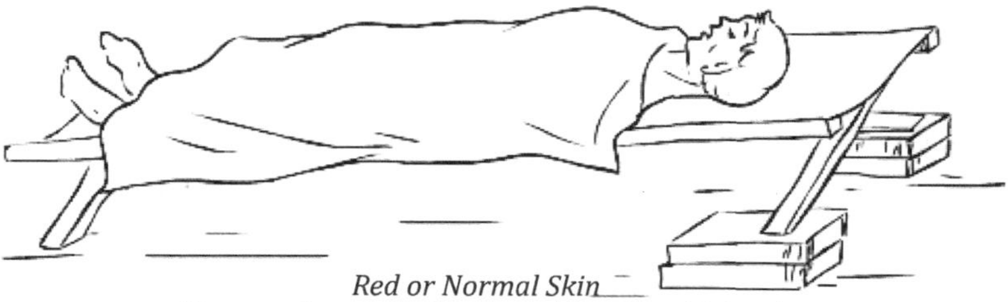

Red or Normal Skin
(Heat stroke, stroke, heart problem, head injury)

WHEN SOMETHING GETS STUCK IN THE THROAT:

Recommended steps

When something gets stuck in a person's throat and he cannot breathe, quickly do this:

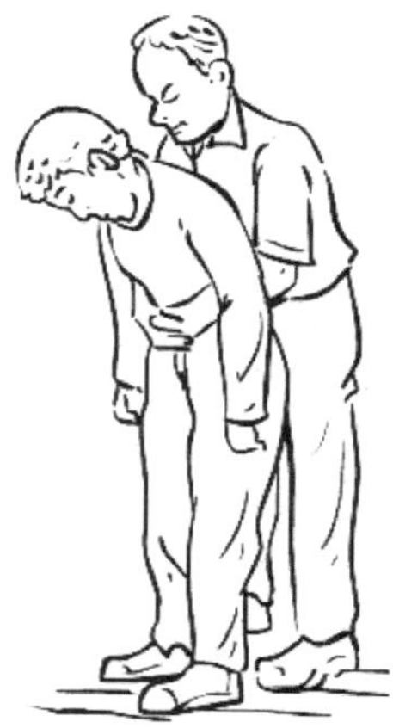

- Stand behind him and wrap your arms around his waist.
- Put your fist against his belly above the naval and below his ribs.
- Now press his belly with a sudden strong upward jerk.
- Repeat several times if necessary.

If the person is lot bigger than you or unconscious do this:

- Lay him on his back.
- Tilt his head to one side.
- Sit over him as shown in picture, with the heel of your lower hand on his belly between his naval and ribs.
- Make a quick, strong upward push.
- Repeat several times if necessary.

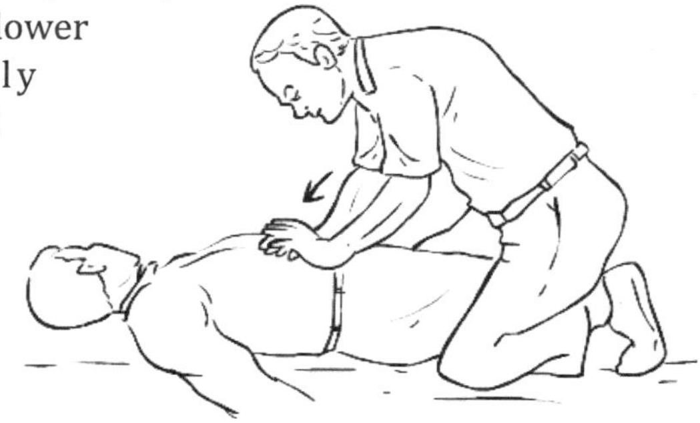

- If he still cannot breathe try mouth to mouth breathing.

DROWNING

Recommended steps

- Always start mouth to mouth breathing at once before trying to get water out of the drowning person's chest.

WHEN BREATHING STOPS, MOUTH TO MOUTH BREATHING:

Common causes for breathing to stop:

- Something stuck in the throat.
- The tongue or thick mucus blocking the throat of an unconscious person.
- Drowning, choking on smoke, or poisoning.
- A strong blow to the head or chest.
- A heart attack.

If a person stops breathing do all of the following as quickly as you can:

- Quickly use a finger to remove anything stuck in the mouth or throat.

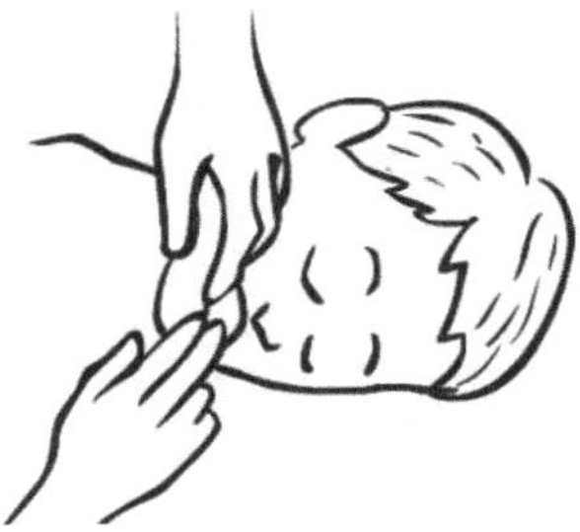

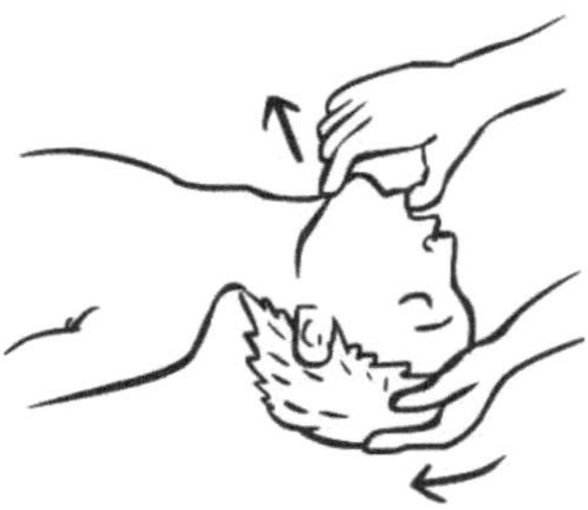

- Quickly but gently lay the person's face up. Gently tilt his head back, and pull his jaw forward.

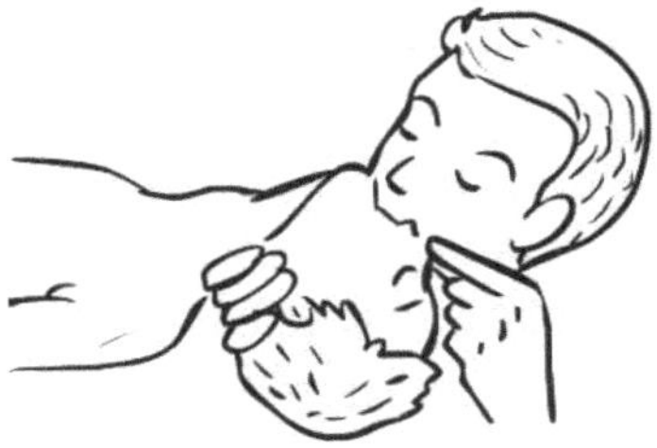

- Pinch his nostrils closed with your fingers, open his mouth wide, cover his mouth with yours and blow strongly into his lungs so that his chest rises. Pause to let the air come back out and blow again. Repeat about once every 5 seconds. With babies and small children, cover the nose and mouth with your mouth and breathe very gently about once every 3 seconds.

EMERGENCIES CAUSED BY HEAT:

Heat Cramps:

- Put a teaspoon of salt in a liter of boiled water and drink it. Repeat once every hour until the cramps are gone.
- Make the person sit or lie down in a cool place and gently message the painful areas.

Differences between 'Heat Exhaustion' and 'Heat Stroke'

Heat Exhaustion

- Sweaty, pale, cool skin
- Large pupils
- No fever

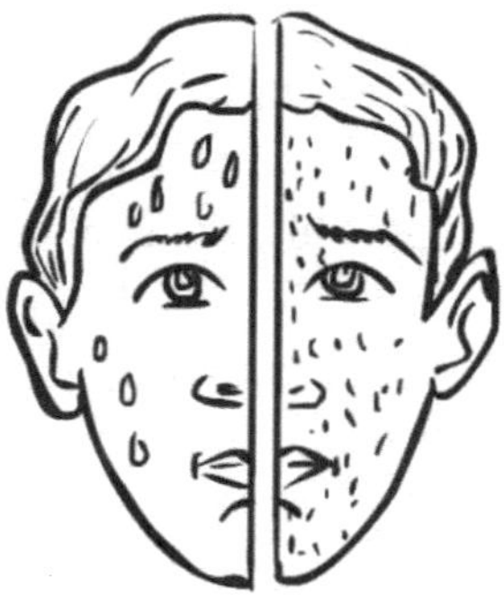

Heat Stroke

- Dry, red, hot skin
- High fever
- The person is very ill or unconscious

Heat Exhaustion:

Recommended steps

- Make the person lie down in a cool place.
- Raise his feet and rub his legs.
- Give salt water to drink.
- Give nothing by mouth while the person is unconscious.

Heat Stroke:

Recommended steps

- The body temperature must be lowered immediately.
- Put the person in the shade.
- Soak him with cold water and fan him.
- Continue until the fever stops.

HOW TO CONTROL BLEEDING FROM A WOUND:

- Raise the injured part.
- Press directly on the wound & keep pressing until the bleeding stops.
- Keep the wounded part as high as possible.
- Maintain the pressure by binding the wound tightly with a bandage or a piece of clean clothing.

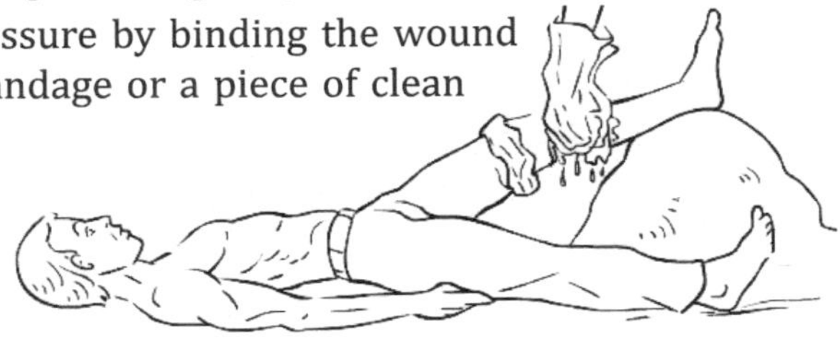

- Squeeze at pressure points on the artery that brings blood to that part of the body.
- Keep pressing for 20 minutes before looking to see if the bleeding has stopped.

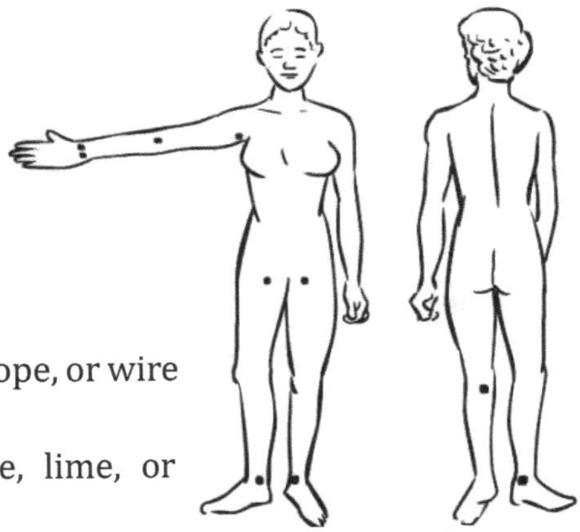

Pressure points

Precautions:

- Do not use a tourniquet, rope, or wire to stop the bleeding.
- Never use dirt, kerosene, lime, or coffee to stop bleeding.
- When bleeding or injury is severe, raise the feet and lower the head to prevent shock.
- Keep blood away from getting into any cuts or sores on your skin.

NOSE BLEEDING

Causes:

- Cold or flu
- Allergies
- Nasal tumor

- Nose injury
- Nasal infection

Symptoms:

- Expelling of blood from the nostril.

How to stop nosebleeds:

- Sit quietly and upright.
- Blow the nose gently to remove mucus and blood.

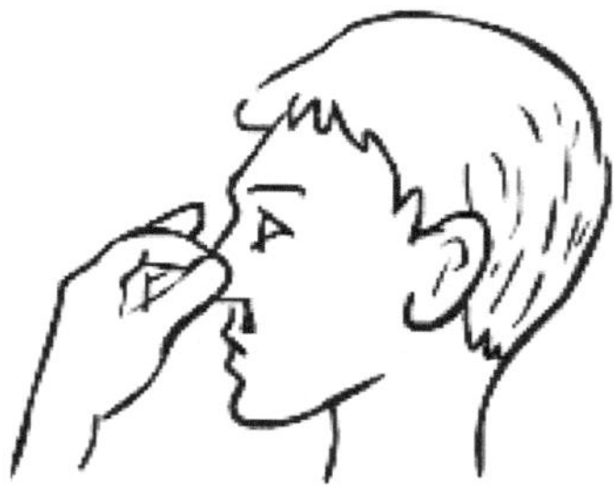

- Let the person pinch the nose firmly for 10 minutes or until the bleeding has stopped.
- Squeeze out some fresh lemon juice. Soak a cotton bud in it and gently dab inside of your nose, leaving part of it outside. Injured blood vessels contract as soon as they come into contact with lemon juice.

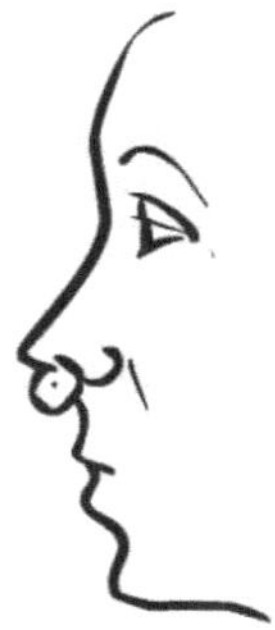

- Do not tip the head back.

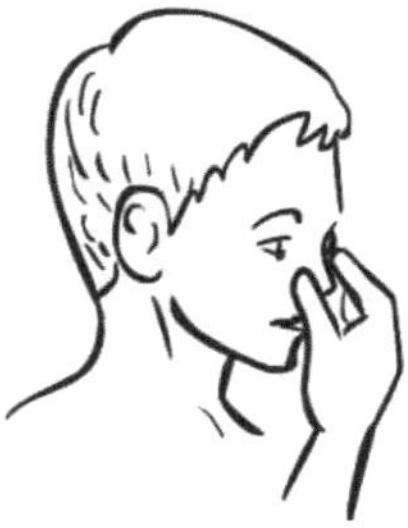

- Leave the cotton in place for a few hours after the bleeding stops, take it out very carefully.
- In older person especially, bleeding may come from the back part of the nose and cannot be stopped by pinching it. In this case, have the person hold a cork, corn cob or

other similar object between his teeth and lean forward, sit quietly and try not to swallow until the bleeding stops.

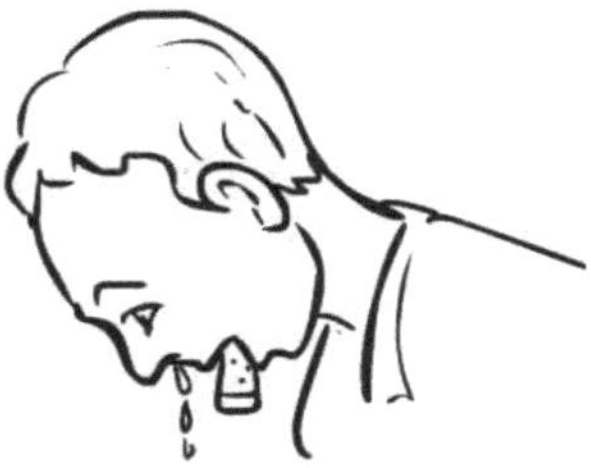

CUTS, SCRAPS AND SMALL WOUNDS

- First wash your hands very well with water.
- If the wound is bleeding or oozing, wear gloves or plastic bag on your hands.
- Wash the skin around the wound with cool, boiled water.
- Lift up and clean under flaps of skin if any.
- If possible squirt out the wound with cool boiled water in a syringe or suction bulb.

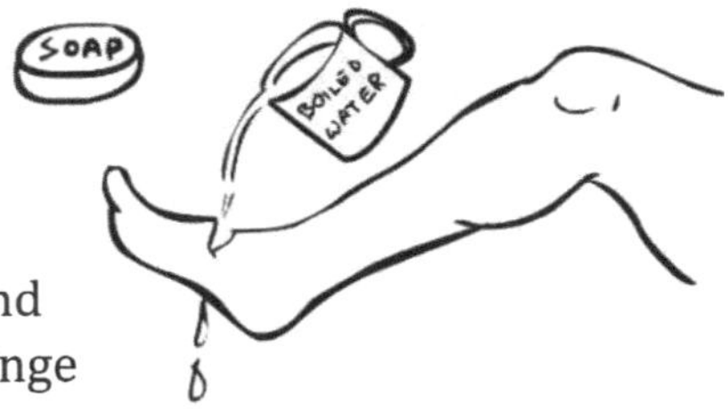

HOW TO CLOSE LARGE CUTS

Bring the edges together and close a deep cut for fast healing if:

- The cut is less than 12 hours old.
- The cut is very clean.
- It is impossible to get a health worker to close it the same day.
- Before closing the cut, wash it very well with cool, boiled water.

BANDAGES

- Bandages must be always clean.
- It is better to have no bandage at all than one that is dirty or wet.
- Change the bandage every day.
- For children it is often better to bandage the whole hand or foot instead of one finger or toe.

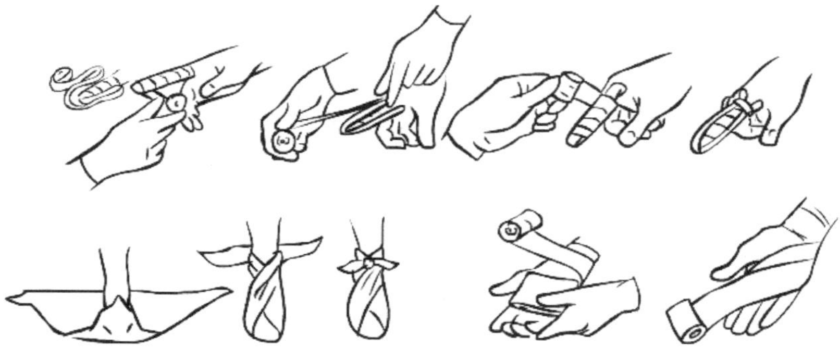

Infected wounds: How to recognize and treat them

Signs & Symptoms:

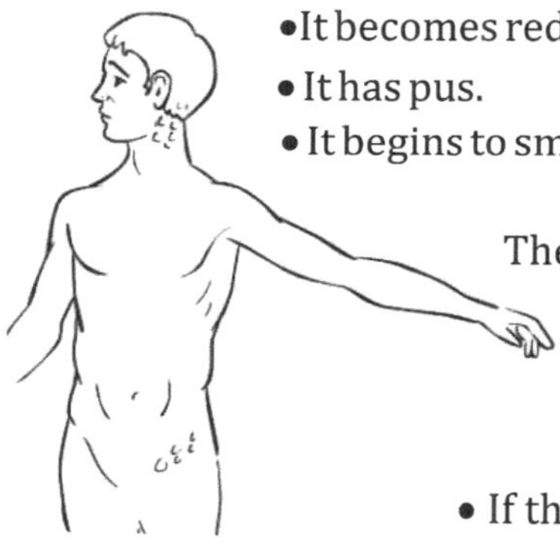

- It becomes red, swollen, hot and painful.
- It has pus.
- It begins to smell bad.

The infection is spreading to other parts of the body if:

- It causes fever.
- There is a red line above the wound.
- If the lymph nodes become swollen and tender.

Treatment of infected wounds:

- Put hot compresses over the wound for 20 minutes 4 times a day. Or hold an infected hand or foot in a bucket of hot water for 20 min.
- Keep the infected part at rest and elevated.

When the wound is serious:

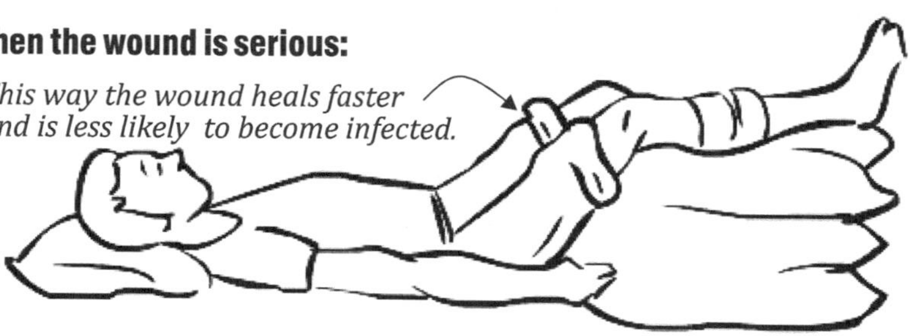

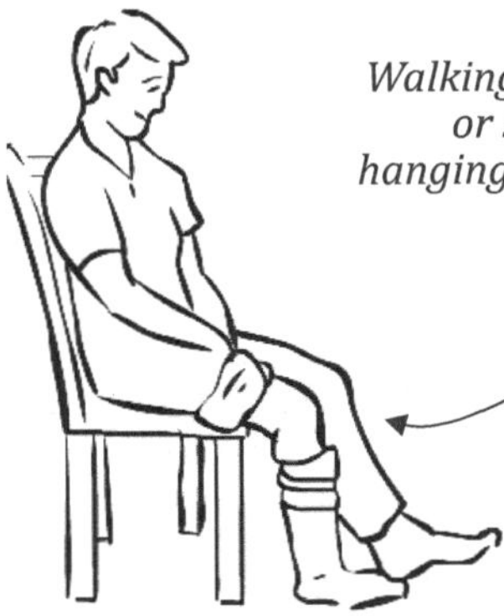

Walking on with an injured leg or sitting with the leg hanging down will slow healing the infection

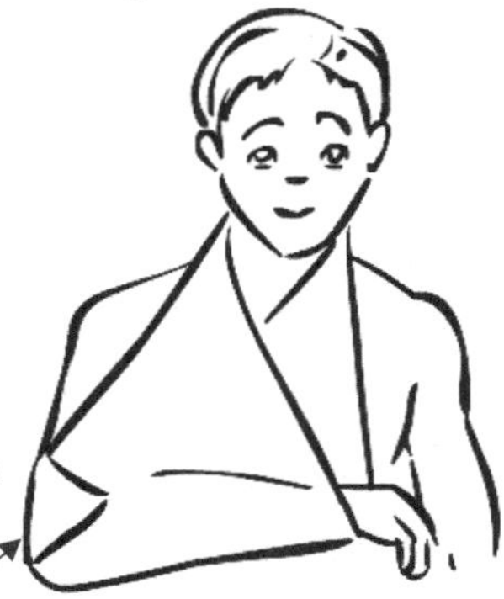

Make a sling like this to support an arm with a gunshot wound or other serious injury.

Deep Chest Wounds:

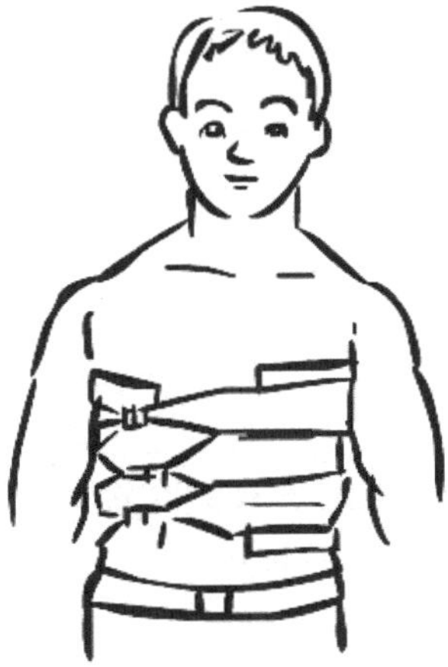

- Cover the wound immediately, if the wound has reached the lungs and air is being sucked through the hole when the person breathes.
- Put the injured person in the position in which he feels most comfortable.
- If there are signs of shock give him proper treatment.

BULLET WOUNDS IN THE HEAD:

Recommended steps

- Place the injured person in half sitting position.
- Cover the wound with the clean bandage.

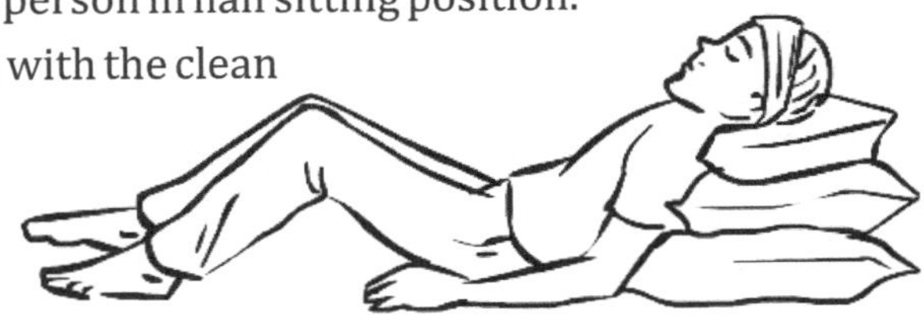

Deep wounds in the abdomen:

Recommended Steps

- Cover the wound with a clean bandage.
- If the guts are partly outside the wound, cover them with a clean cloth soaked in lightly salted, cool, boiled water.
- Don not try to push the guts back in.
- If the wounded person is in shock, raise his feet higher than his head.
- Give absolutely nothing by mouth.
- If the wounded person is awake and thirsty, let him suck on a piece of cloth soaked in water.
- Never give him enema, even if the stomach swells up or the injured person does not move his bowels for days.

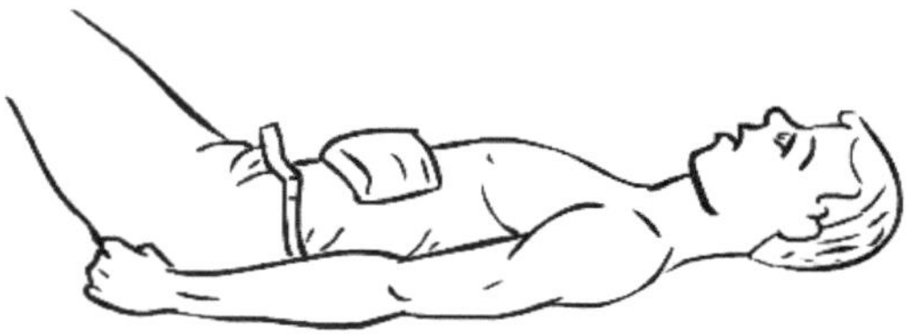

BURNS

First degree burns:

- Involve outer layer of the skin only.
- Painful and redness like sunburn.

Second degree burns:

- Extends to middle skin layer.
- Redness, swollen and blistering.

Recommended steps

First and second degree burns:

- Get away from the heat source.
- Cool the burnt area under running cold water continuously for 10 minutes.
- Or damp the burnt area with a towel soaked in cold water.
- Apply a solution of Tulsi (Basil) leaves juice and coconut oil to alleviate pain.

- For burns from hot liquid rub the affected area with ice cube and then apply a solution of milk and honey
- Sliced potatoes can also be used on an affected area for relief.
- Apply Aloe Vera gel to ease burns, relieve inflammation and accelerate healing.

BROKEN BONES (FRACTURES)

- Keep the bones in a fixed position.
- When trying to move or carry a person with broken bones, keep the bones from moving with splints, strips of bark, a sleeve of cardboard.

Setting broken bones: If the bones are far out of position and the break is recent, try to set or straighten them before putting on cast.

How to set a broken wrist:

Step 1: Pull the hand with a slow, steady force for 5 to 10 minutes; increase the force to separate the bones.

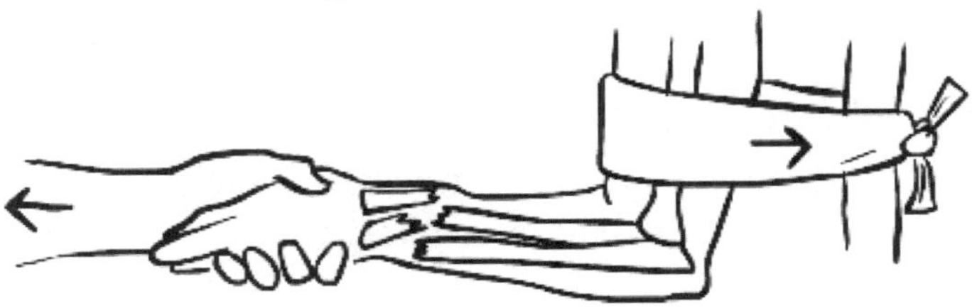

Step 2: With one person still pulling the hand, have another gently line up and straighten up the bones.

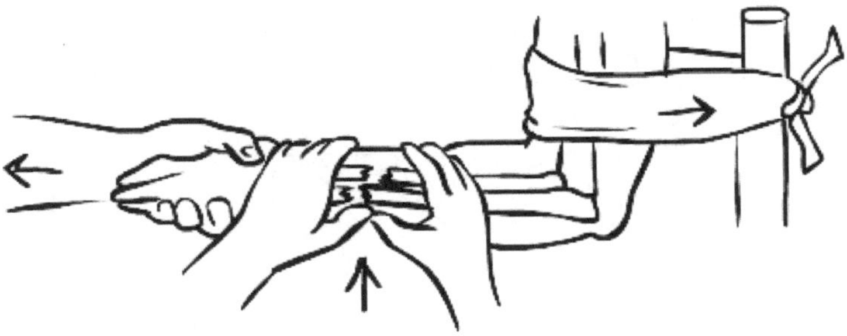

Note: It is possible to do a lot of damage while trying to set a bone. Ideally, it should be done with the help of someone with experience. Do not jerk or force.

How long does it take for broken bones to heal?

- The older the person, the longer the healing takes.
- Children's bones mend rapidly.
- A broken arm should be kept in a cast for about a month, and no force put on it for another month.
- A broken leg should remain in a cast for about 2 months.

DISLOCATIONS

Recommended Steps:

- Try to put the bone back into place. The sooner the better.
- Keep it bandaged firmly in place so it does not slip out again.
- Avoid forceful use of the limb long enough for the joint to heal completely (2 or 3 months).

How to set a dislocated shoulder:

- Make the injured person lie face down on a table or other firm surface with his arm hanging over the side.

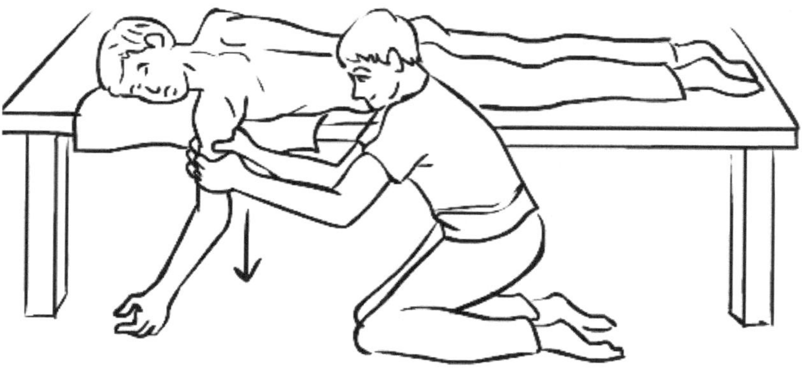

- Pull down on the arm towards the floor, using a strong steady force, for 15 to 20 minutes. Then gently let it go.
- The shoulder should pop back into place.
- Or attach something to the arm that weighs 10 to 20 lbs and leave it there for 15 to 20 minutes.
- After the shoulder is in place, bandage the arm firmly against the body.
- Keep it bandaged for a week to a month.

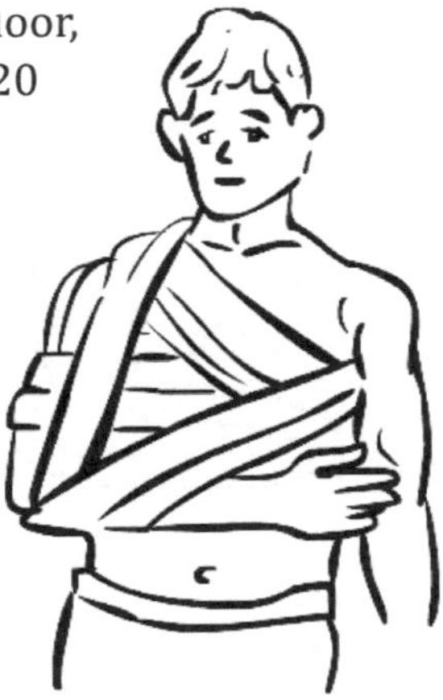

- To prevent the shoulder from becoming completely stiff, unbandage the arm for a few minutes for three times a day and with the arm hanging at the side, move it gently in narrow circles.
- Do not lift any weight with the arm for a month so that the shoulder does not pop out of the place again.

STRAINS AND SPRAINS

Signs & Symptoms:

- Pain
- Swelling
- Bruises or redness.
- Inability to move the injured part.

Recommended steps:

- Keep the joint motionless.
- Wrap it with something that gives firm support.
- Use crutches to give a sprained foot as much rest as possible.
- To relieve pain and swelling, elevate the injured part.
- Put ice wrapped in cloth or put plastic over the swollen joint for 20 to 30 minutes once in every hour.

- After 24 to 48 hours soak the sprain in hot water for several times a day.

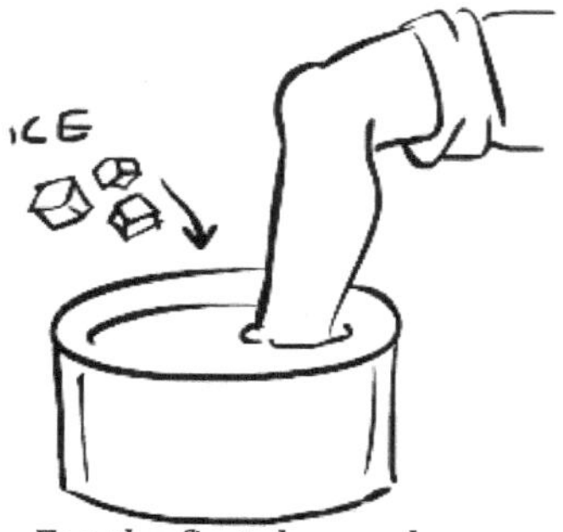

For the first day soak the sprained joint in cold water

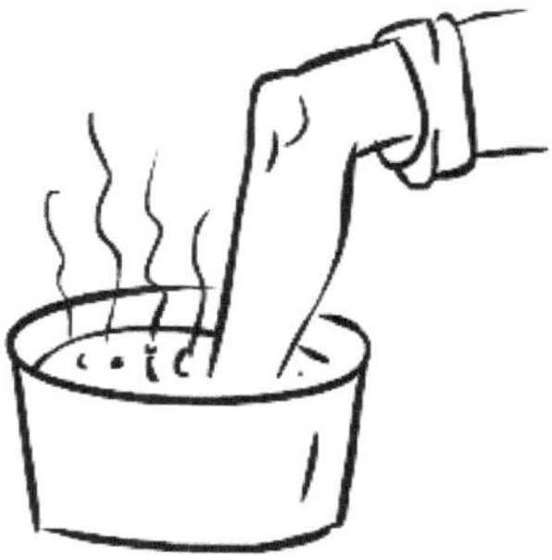

After 1 or 2 days use hot soaks.

- Wrapping the foot and ankle with an elastic bandage will also prevent or reduce swelling.
- Never rub or massage a sprain or broken bone.

FAINTING

Signs & symptoms:

- Giddiness and nausea.
- Excessive sweating.
- Blurred vision.
- Rapid heartbeat.
- Pale and clammy skin.
- Loss of consciousness and falling down.

Recommended steps:

- Lay the victim down on his or her back.
- If he vomits turn him onto his side.
- Loosen the tight clothing.
- If the victim has fallen, look for injuries.
- Do not splash or pour water on the victim's face.

- Do not use smelling salts or ammonia inhalants.
- Do not slap the victim's face as an attempt to revive him or her.
- Do not give the victim anything to drink until he or she has fully recovered.

HEALING WITH WATER

Prevention

To help prevent	Use water
1. Diarrhea, worms, gut infections	Boil or filter drinking water, wash hands etc.
2. Skin infections	Bathe often
3. Wounds becoming infected, tetanus	Wash wounds well with soap and clean water

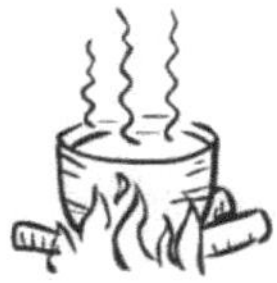

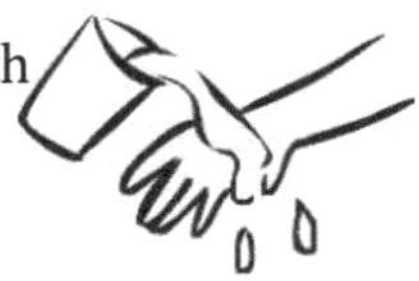

TREATMENT

To Treat	Use Water
1. Diarrhea, dehydration	Drink plenty of liquids.
2. Illness with fever High fever	Drink plenty of liquids Remove clothing and soak body with cool water.
3. Minor urinary infections	Drink plenty of water.
4. Cough, asthma, bronchitis, pneumonia, whooping cough	Drink a lot of water and breathe hot water vapors to loosen mucus.

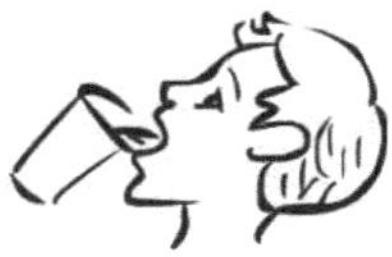

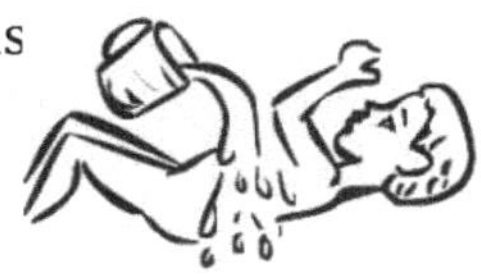

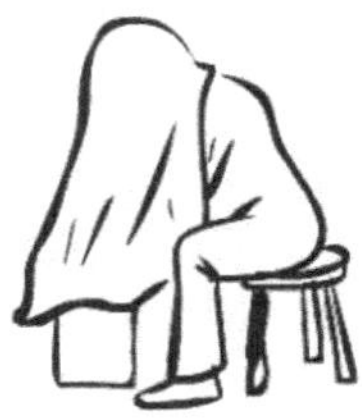

To Treat	Use Water	
5. Sores, impetigo, ring worm of skin or scalp, cradle cap, pimples	Scrub with clean water.	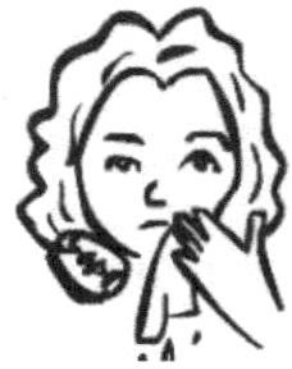
6. Infected wounds, abscesses, boils	Hot soaks or compresses.	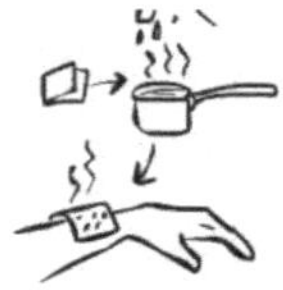
7. Strains and sprains	The first day soak joint in cold water then use hot soaks.	
8. Itching, burning or weeping irritations of the skin	Cold compresses	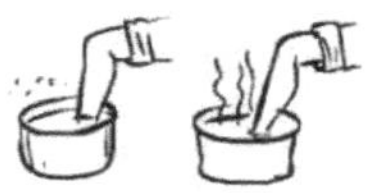
9. Minor burns	Hold in cold water at once.	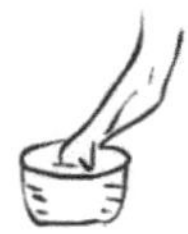
10. Sore throat or tonsillitis	Gargle with warm salt water.	
11. Acid, lye, dirt or irritating substance in eye	Flood eye with cool water at once, and continue for 30 minutes.	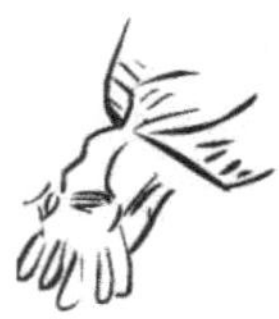
12. Stuffed up nose	Sniff salt water.	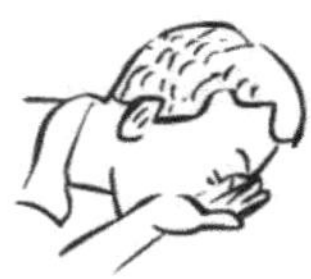
Constipation, hard stools	Drink lots of water.	
13. Cold sores or fever blisters	Hold ice on blister for 1 hr at first sign.	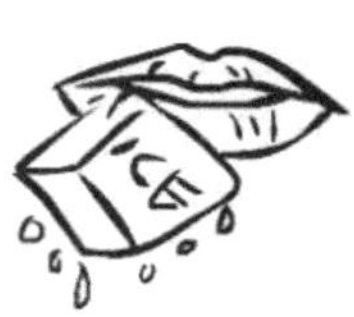

Note:

Note:

SECTION III

This section is dedicated to cure some common sicknesses. Here you will learn drug free methods which will help a patient to recover quickly from the illness without the side effects of the conventional drug induced treatments.

SOME VERY COMMON SICKNESSES

DEHYDRATION

Symptoms:

- Thirst is often a first, early sign of dehydration.
- Little or no urine, the urine is dark yellow.
- Sudden weight loss.
- Dry mouth.
- Sunken, tearless eyes.
- **Sagging in** of the 'soft spot' in infants.
- Loss of elasticity or stretchiness of the skin.

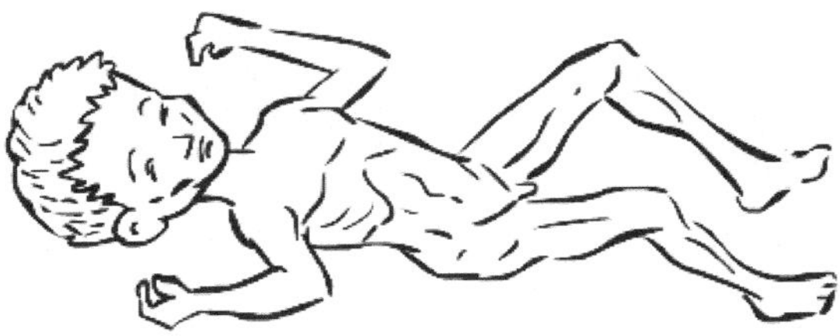

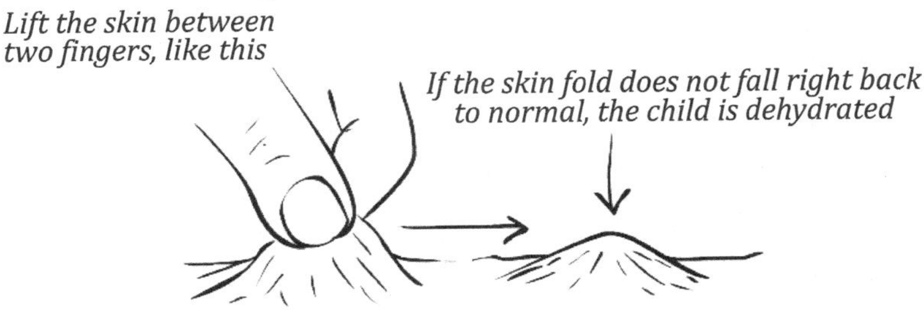

Cure:

- Drink Lemon juice and honey 5 - 6 times a day.

Juice Therapy:

- Watermelon juice
- Lime juice
- Drink a mixture of 1 tsp mint juice, 1/2 tsp Ginger juice and 1 tsp honey 3 times a day.

DIARRHEA

Main causes of Diarrhea

- Poor nutrition
- Shortage of water and unclean conditions
- Virus infection
- Gut infection
- Worm infections
- Malaria
- Food poisoning
- HIV
- Allergies to certain foods
- Laxatives, purges, irritating or poisonous plants
- Eating too much unripe fruits

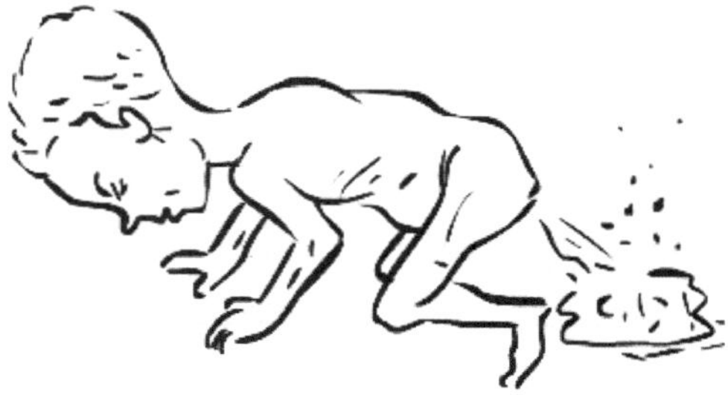

The vicious circle of malnutrition and diarrhea takes many children's lives.

Symptoms:

- Anemic and pale face
- Abdominal pain
- Nausea and vomiting

Cure:

- Mix little salt in lemon and drink without diluting.
- Swallow 25 grams of powdered tulsi seeds with 10 ml honey.

Juice Therapy:

- Drink carrot juice.
- Drink coconut water.
- Drink potato juice mixed with carrot and pure honey.

VOMITING

- Stomach upset
- Mild stomach or gut ache or fever.
- Over eating
- Ingestion of toxins or excessive amounts of alcohol.

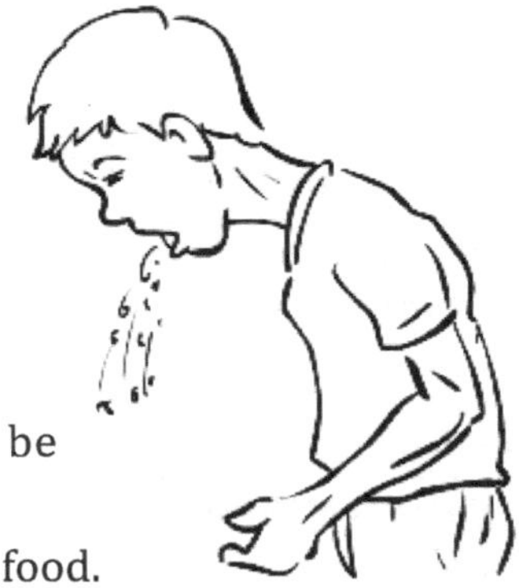

Cure:

- Drink plenty of water.
- Juices and soft drinks should be avoided.
- Eat as tolerated, but only light, bland food.
- Stay away from fried or greasy food.
- Eat small meals and eat them slowly.
- Rest a while after eating with your head elevated.

HEADACHES AND MIGRAINES

Symptoms:

- Severe throbbing headache at one side of the head only.
- Blurring of vision.
- Seeing strange spots of light.
- Numbness of one hand or foot.

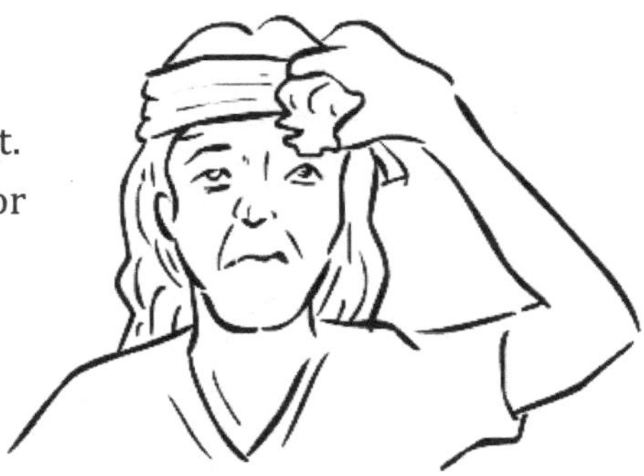

Cure:

- Drink lots of water.
- Massage aloe vera gel over the head.
- Apply fine paste of cinnamon mixed with water on forehead.

Juice Therapy:

- Drink 50 ml of grape juice in the morning for 15 days.
- Drink celery juice.

COLD AND FLU

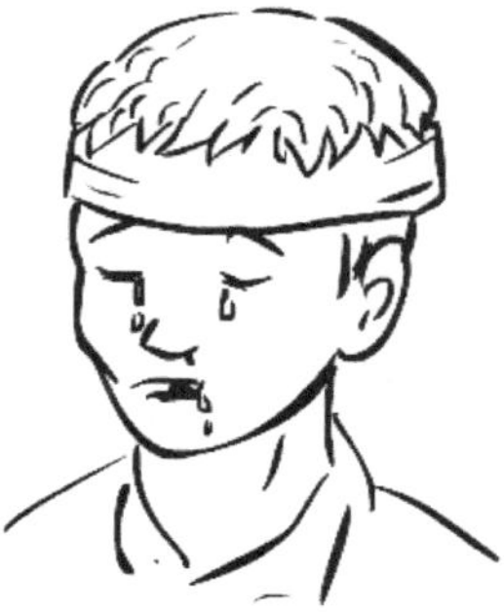

Symptoms:

- Runny nose & cough.
- Sore throat, and sometimes fever or pain in joints.

Cure:

- Eat one amla twice a day.
- Drink mixture of 2 teaspoon of tulsi juice, 2 tsp of ginger juice and honey.

Juice Therapy:

- Drink orange juice.
- Drink mixed vegetables juice.

STUFFY AND RUNNY NOSES

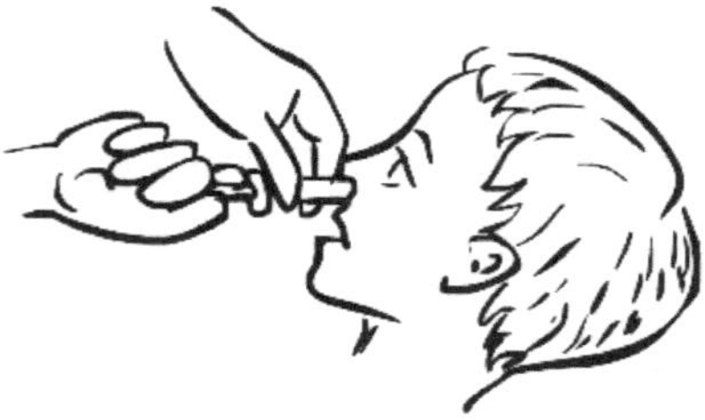

Symptoms:

- Mucus in the nose.
- Ear infection in children.
- Sinus problem in adults.

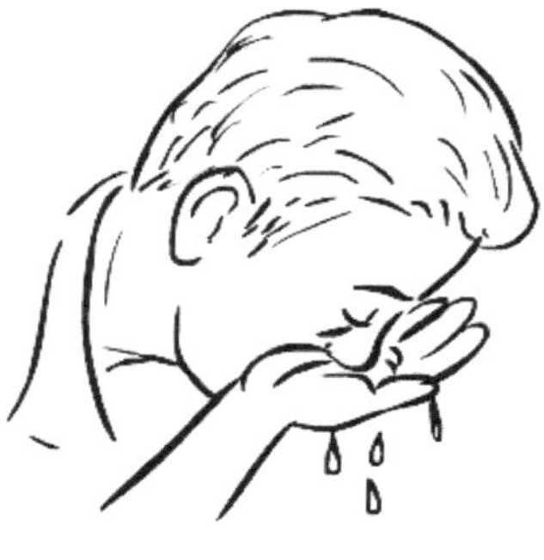

Cure:

- In children, carefully stuck the mucus out of nose with suction bulb.
- Sniff salt water into the nose.
- Breathe hot water vapors.

SINUS TROUBLE (SINUSITIS)

Symptoms:

- Pain in the face above and below the eyes.
- Thick mucus or pus in the nose.
- Fever

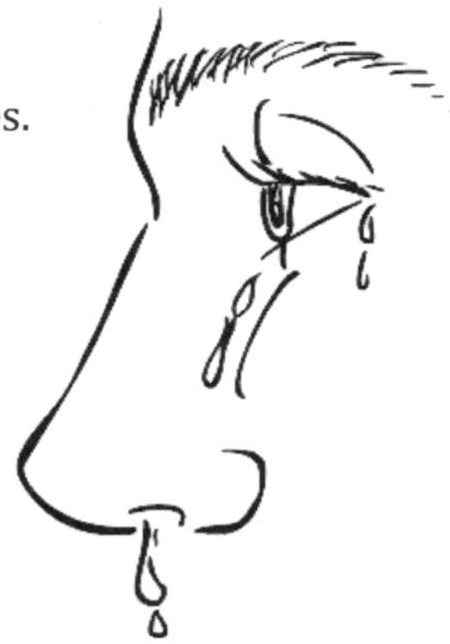

Cure:

- Drink a lot of water.
- Sniff a little salt water into the nose.
- Put hot compresses on the face.

HAY FEVER

Symptoms:

- A runny nose.
- A constant "tickly feeling" in the nose.
- Repeated and prolonged sneezing fits.
- Red, swollen, and itchy eyes that water constantly.
- An itchy throat caused by nasal drainage.
- A stuffy nose.

Cure:

- Gargle with warm salt water.
- Increase the intake of raw honey in your diet.
- Wear a dust mask when doing outdoor activities such as gardening.
- Eat diet rich in Vitamin C.

ASTHMA

Symptoms:

- Hissing or wheezing sound when breathing out.
- Skin goes behind the collar bones.

- Ribs may suck.
- Nails and lips may turn blue.
- Neck veins may swell.

Cure:

- Mix the juice of one clove of garlic with 1 tsp of honey and drink it twice a day.
- Mix 1 tsp tulsi juice and 1 tsp honey and drink it 3 times a day.

Juice Therapy:

- Drink apple juice
- Drink lemon juice
- Drink 20 ml of carrot juice daily

COUGH

Causes:

Dry Cough with little or no phlegm	Cough with much or little phlegm	Cough with a wheeze or whoop and trouble breathing
• Cold or flu • Worms - when passing through lungs • Measles • Smoking	• Bronchitis • Pneumonia • Asthma • Smoking	• Asthma • Whooping cough • Diphtheria • Heart trouble • Something stuck in the throat

Chronic or persistent cough	Coughing up blood
• Tuberculosis • Smoker's or minor's cough • Asthma • Chronic bronchitis • Emphysema	• Tuberculosis • Pneumonia • Severe worm infection • Cancer of lungs or throat

Symptoms:

- Thick yellow or green phlegm.

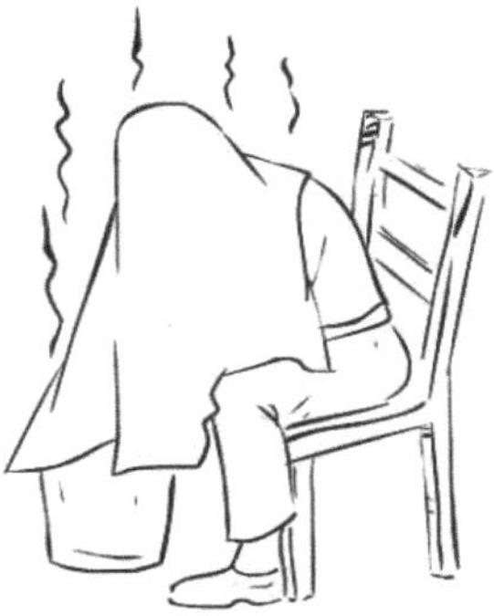

Cure

- Drink lots of water.
- Breathe hot water vapors.
- Mix 5 ml onion juice with 10 ml honey and drink it twice a day for 10 days.
- Boil some basil leaves in water and drink this every morning.
- Mix equal amount of honey and ginger juice and drink 1 tsp 2 -3 times a day.
- For dry cough the following cough syrup can be given:

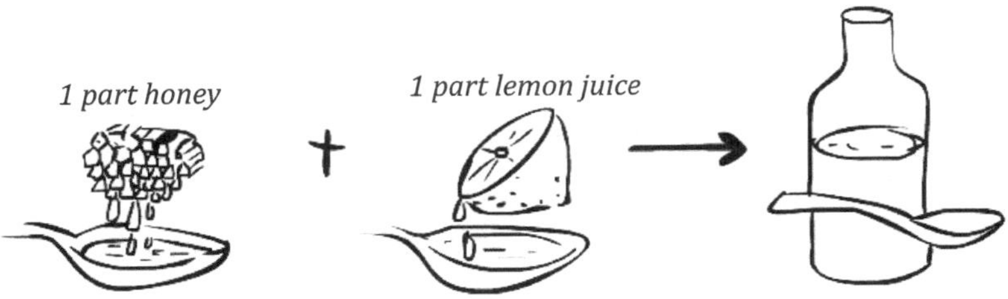

Juice Therapy:

- Drink 1 cup of grape juice mixed with 1 tsp of honey.
- Drink 1 tsp of onion juice mixed with 1 tsp of honey.
- For severe cough, fast on orange juice and water.

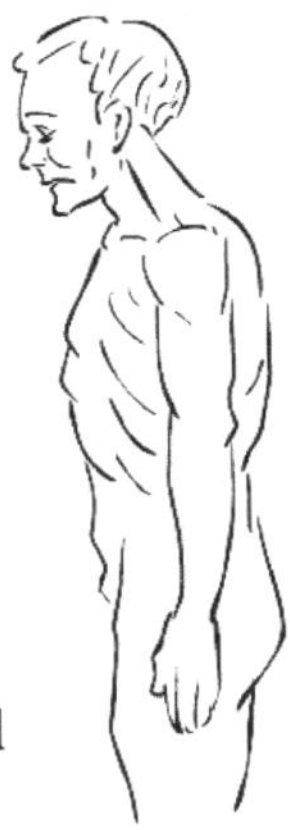

BRONCHITIS

Symptoms:

- Noisy cough.
- Mucus or phlegm.
- Chest pain or tightening of chest.
- Fever, muscle ache, nasal congestion, and tiredness.

Cure:

- Staying well hydrated by drinking fluids.
- Drink orange juice.
- Avoid dairy products, alcohol and caffeine.
- If the person has trouble coughing up sticky phlegm, make him breathe hot water vapors.
- Stop smoking.

PNEUMONIA

Symptoms:

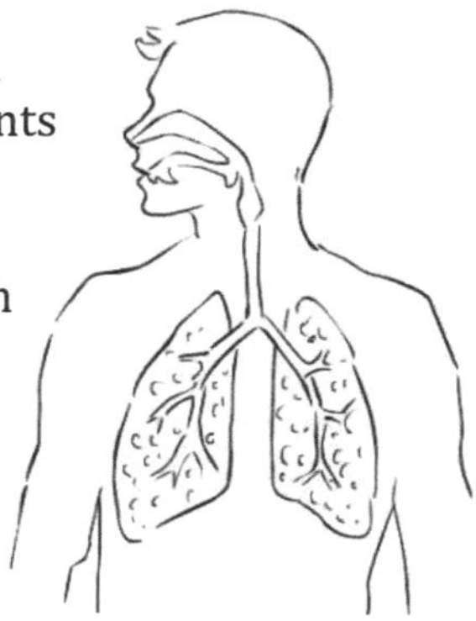

- Sudden chills and then high fever.
- Rapid, shallow breathing, with little grunts or sometimes wheezing.
- Fever
- Cough (often with yellow greenish, rush colored or slightly bloody mucus).
- Chest pain.
- A cold sore often appears on the face or lips.

Cure:

- Take plenty of rest.
- Drink plenty of fluids, especially water to help loosen mucus in your lungs.
- Take steam bath.
- Increase intake of ginger and garlic.
- Consume a mixture of 100 ml of carrot juice and 100 ml of cucumber juice once in a day.

HEPATITIS

Symptoms:

- Feels tired.
- Pain on the right side near the liver.
- Fever

- Eyes turn yellow.
- Sight or smell of food may cause vomiting.
- Urine may turn dark like Coca Cola, and the stools become whitish.

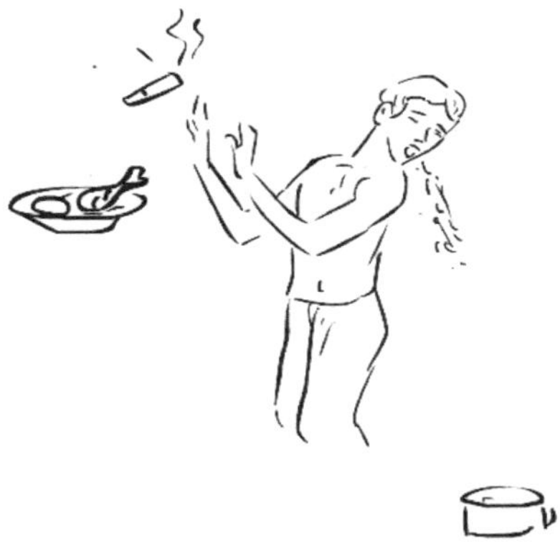

Cure:

- Drink mixture of 2 tsp of coriander leaves juice.
- Drink aloe vera juice.

Juice therapy:

- Drink beetroot and carrot juice daily.
- Drink wheatgrass juice.

ARTHRITIS (PAINFUL, INFLAMED JOINTS)

Causes:

- Inability to produce endorphin.
- Joint injuries & infections.
- Stress and Sprain.

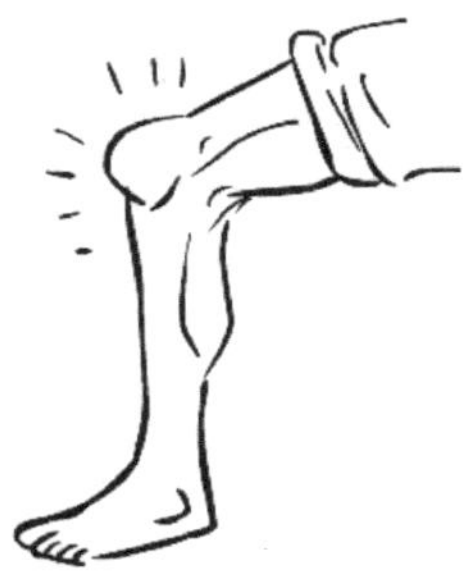

Symptoms:

- Inflammation of the joints.
- Deformity of joints.
- Swelling of joints.

Cure:

- Eat 1-2 garlic cloves on an empty stomach every morning.
- Squeeze half lemon in one glass of hot water and drink 2-3 times a day.
- Drink 50 ml of amla juice for 4 weeks with an empty stomach.

Juice Therapy:

- Drink black cherry juice twice a day.
- Drink apple juice.
- Drink potato juice.

BACK PAIN

Causes:

- Weak abdominal and back muscles.
- Wearing high heels.
- Long hours of sitting.
- Standing or sitting with the shoulder drooped.
- Lifting heavy loads in an incorrect way.
- In older people, the chronic back pain is often arthritis.
- Pain in the upper right back may be from a gallbladder problem.
- Very low back pain sometimes comes from the problems in the uterus, ovaries or rectum.

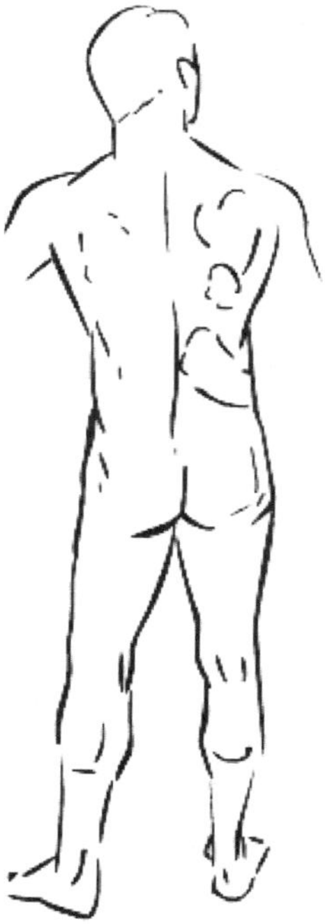

Symptoms:

- Pain in the middle of the back or in the lower back
- In acute stage, the patient is bed ridden and unable to move.

Cure:

- Boil water with tulsi leaves and black cardamom and drink.
- Apply Aloe Vera gel on back.

Juice Therapy:

- Drink lemon juice
- Drink cherry juice

VARICOSE VEINS

- Veins swollen, twisted, and often painful.
- Fatigue, restlessness, and feelings of burning throbbing, tingling, or heaviness in the legs.

Cure:

- Do not spend much time with standing or sitting with your feet down.
- Avoid sugar, ice cream, fried foods, junk foods, cheese, tobacco, salt, alcohol, and processed and refined foods.
- Exercise daily.
- Do not wear tight clothes.
- Avoid standing or sitting for long period of time.
- Avoid scratching the itchy skin above varicose veins.
- Use elastic stockings or elastic bandages to help hold in the veins.

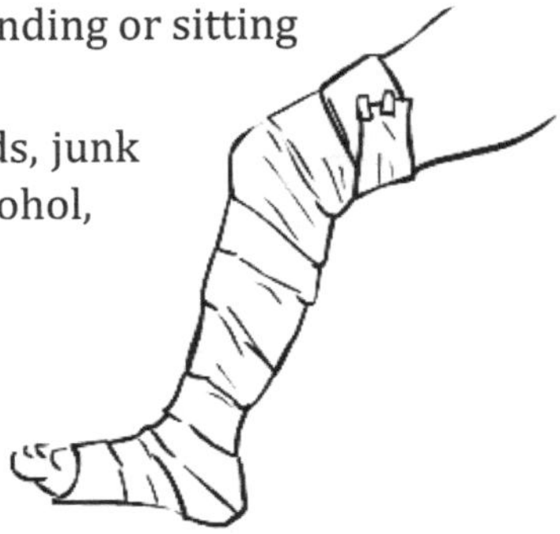

PILES (HEMORRHOIDS)

Causes:

- Persistent constipation.
- Prolonged periods of standing or sitting.
- Strenuous work.
- Obesity
- General weakness of the tissues of the body.
- Mental tension.
- Heredity

Symptoms:

- Pain while passing stools.
- Slight bleeding in the case of internal trouble.

- Feeling of soreness and irritation after passing stool.
- Discomfort around the rectal area.

Cure:

- Eat raw onions.
- Or mix paste of onion with ginger and eat twice a day for 7 days.
- Consume aloe vera juice

Juice Therapy:

- Drink 100 ml turnip leaves juice twice daily.
- Drink radish juice.
- Mix 1/2 tsp of ginger juice, 1 tsp of lime juice and 1 tsp of mint juice with honey and drink once in a day.

SWELLING OF THE FEET AND OTHER PARTS OF THE BODY

Causes:

- Overweight
- Old age
- Pregnancy
- Leg infection
- Diabetes
- Injury of the leg, ankle or feet.
- Varicose veins have been troubling you (for quite some time).
- Intake of diet with too much salt (sodium).
- Sunburn or burns on your feet.

Cure:

- Do not spend time sitting with your feet down.
- When you sit, put your feet up high.
- While sleeping, make sure your feet are raised.
- Take breaks often to stand up and move around.

- Try cutting back on salt. This will reduce the buildup of fluids in your feet.
- Soak your feet in warm concentrated salt water for a while.

HERNIA (RUPTURE)

Causes:

- Lifting heavy objects.
- Obesity
- Persistent coughing.
- Strain while urinating or during bowel movements.
- Chronic lung disease.
- Accumulation of fluid in the abdominal cavity.
- Family history of hernias.

Symptoms:

- Loss of Appetite
- Pain
- Pressure in lower abdomen.
- Swelling
- Lump near belly button.

Cure:

- Ice compresses are one of the best home remedies for hernia.
- Avoid applying any heat or pressure to the affected area.
- Avoid exercising on a full stomach.
- Avoid eating large meals and opt for smaller, frequent meals throughout the day.
- Refrain from lying down or bending soon after eating.
- Avoid consuming alcohol.
- Tight clothes can exert pressure on the abdomen and hence it is advisable to wear only loose, comfortable clothing.

EPILEPSY

Causes:

- Injury to baby during delivery.
- Delay in delivery with decreased oxygen supply.
- Excessive fluid in the brain.

Symptoms:

- Patient loses control over passing of urine and stool.
- Headache after gaining consciousness.
- Sudden spasms of head and trunk.

Cure:

- Apply lemon juice on head.
- Boil 3-4 crushed garlic cloves with 100 ml milk & drink it when it is reduced to half.
- After taking bath, rub tulsi juice over the body.

Juice Therapy:

- Consume 20-30 ml of wheat grass juice daily on an empty stomach.

HIGH CHOLESTEROL

Causes:

- Excessive consumption of milk and its products like ghee, butter and cream.
- Fried food and oily food.
- Irregularity in habits, smoking, drinking alcohols.

Symptoms:

- High cholesterol doesn't have any symptom, for that you go through a simple blood test called a Lipoprotein Profile.

Cure:

- Drink at least 8 to 10 glasses of water every day.
- Regular drinking of coriander is beneficial.
- Increase the intake of raw garlic.
- Increase the intake of Aloe Vera juice.

Juice Therapy:

- Drink beetroot juice.
- Consume lemon juice and 1 tsp honey in a glass of luke warm water with empty stomach in morning and at night.

INDIGESTION

Causes:

- Eating too fast, especially high fat food.
- Excessive acid accumulation in the stomach.
- Over consumption of alcohol.
- Stress during pregnancy.

Symptoms:

- Burning sensation in stomach or chest.
- Bloating, nausea and burping.

Cure:

- Eat 2 -3 small pieces of ginger before eating heavy meal.
- Mix1 tsp of ginger juice and 1 tsp of lemon juice . Honey can be added according to taste.
- Drink 1 glass of hot water mixed with 2 tsp ginger juice and 1 tsp honey.

HAIR FALL

Causes:

- Inadequate nutrition.
- Deficiency of vitamin and folic acid.
- Stress, worry and anxiety .

Symptoms:

- Thinning of hair.
- Constant shedding of hair .

Cure:

- Cut a lemon into two halves and massage the scalp. After half an hour rinse the hair with cold water.

Juice therapy:

- Drink broccoli and carrot juice.

INFLAMMATION OF GUMS

- Poor oral hygiene.
- Not cleaning mouth after intake of food.

Symptoms:

- Difficulty while chewing food.
- Bleeding and pain in gums.
- Teeth fall out one by one.

Cure:

- Apply garlic paste on the affected tooth.
- Chew tulsi leaves after meal.

Juice Therapy:

- Drink cranberry juice.
- Wheat grass juice is quite helpful in preventing bacterial growth.

JAUNDICE:

Causes:

- Stones in liver.
- Blockage in the pathway of bile.
- Contaminated food and water.
- Certain vitamins deficiency.
- Liver malfunctioning.

Symptoms:

- Yellow complexion
- Nausea
- Fatigue and itching
- Slow pulse
- Yellow eyes
- Loss of appetite

Cure:

- Frequently drink lemon juice.
- Drink wheat grass juice.
- 1 tsp ginger juice with 1 tsp fresh lime juice and tulsi juice mixed with 1 tsp honey should be taken frequently.

Juice Therapy:

- Drink sugarcane juice mixed with the juice of half a lime twice daily.
- Drink tomato juice.

KIDNEY STONE

Causes:

- Defects in the general metabolism.
- Insufficient intake of fluids.
- Excess intake of acid forming foods

Symptoms:

- Obstruction of flow of urine and pain.

- A desire to urinate frequently.
- Painful urination.
- Scanty urination.

Cure:

- Frequent intake of coriander tea.
- Consume basil juice mixed with honey.

Juice Therapy:

- Drink coconut water.
- Drink watermelon juice.
- Drink lemon juice.
- Banana pulp juice also helps in removing kidney stones.

HEART PROBLEM

Causes:

- Excessive smoking.
- Hypertension
- Increased blood cholesterol level.
- Diabetes
- Lack of exercise.
- Excessive alcohol consumption.

Symptoms:

- Pain in chest either on the left, centre or even on the right side.
- Difficulty in breathing .
- Sweating is seen in acute attacks.
- Irregular heartbeat, may be seen in some cases.

Cure:

- One clove of garlic should be taken daily on empty stomach.

- Consume 1 tsp of raw onion juice daily first thing in the morning.
- Take 1 tsp of honey daily after meal.

Juice Therapy:
- Drink 50 ml beet root juice daily.
- Drink freshly prepared grape juice.
- Drink apple juice.

OBESITY

Causes:
- Eating too much.
- Inherited one.
- Result of hormonal disorder.

Symptoms:
- Extra accumulated fat on joints of hips, knees, ankles.
- Coronary thrombosis, heart failure.

Cure:
- Add 1 tsp of honey and fresh juice of half lemon to one glass of lukewarm water and drink twice or thrice a day.

Juice Therapy:
- Drink pineapple juice.
- Drink Aloe Vera juice.

BAD BREATH

Symptoms:
- Odorous breath.
- An unpleasant taste in the mouth.

Cure:
- Chew 4 or 5 tulsi leaves two to four times a day.

- Drink water throughout the day to keep your mouth moistened.
- Chew a little amount of wheat grass for 3 to 5 minutes a day.

Juice Therapy:

- Drink pineapple juice daily.
- Drink apple juice.
- Drink wheat grass juice.

CATARACT

Causes:

- Malnutrition
- Vitamin A or B deficiency
- Diabetes
- Old age
- Infection of an eye.

Symptoms:

- Blurring of vision in the early stages of the disease.
- Complete vision is impaired in the affected eye at later stage.

Cure:

- Mix1 tsp of rose water with 1 tsp fresh lemon juice . Put 1 drop twice or thrice to the affected eye.

Juice Therapy:

- Drink carrot juice.
- Drink juices rich in beta - carotene and vitamin C.

INTESTINAL WORMS

Causes:

- Undercooked meat.
- Dirty fingers and food.
- Through the skin from infected water.
- Undercooked flesh food or foods contaminated by dogs.

Symptoms:

- Diarrhea
- Foul smell
- Dark circles under eyes
- Constant desire for food
- Loss of weight
- Nervousness and irritability

Cure:

- Increase the intake of garlic in your diet.
- Drink aloe vera juice.

Juice Therapy:

- Drink pumpkin juice.
- Drink 1 tsp mint juice three times a day.

IRREGULAR BLEEDING

Causes:

- Imbalance of hormones
- Tension
- Cancer of the uterus

Symptoms:

- Pain in lower abdomen.
- Pain in the lumber and hip region.
- Weakness and giddiness.
- Breathlessness
- Palpitation and anemia.

Cure:

- Eat amla daily.

- Apiece of ginger grounded and boiled in a cup of water should be taken three times a day after meals.

Juice Therapy:

- Drink grape juice daily.
- Drink a carrot juice daily.
- Drink bitter guard juice.

DENGUE

Symptoms:

- High fever, up to 105F.
- Severe headache, backache or both.
- Plain behind your eyes.
- Severe joint and muscle pain.
- Nausea and vomiting.

Causes:

- Blood vessel fluid (plasma) leakage.
- Heavy bleeding.
- A sudden drop in blood pressure.

Cure:

- Drink lots of water.
- Chew 10 - 15 basil leaves twice a day.

Juice Therapy:

- Drink 20 ml raw papaya leaf juice twice a day.
- Drink orange juice.
- Drink wheat grass juice.

Note:

Note:

SECTION IV

This section focuses on the life style oriented diseases which make the patients drug dependent for their entire life time and in most of the cases these drugs are very expensive. The simple strategies given in this section will help a patient to recover from the lifestyle diseases permanently.

SERIOUS ILLNESSES THAT NEED SPECIAL MEDICAL ATTENTION

TUBERCULOSIS (TB)

Most Common Symptoms:

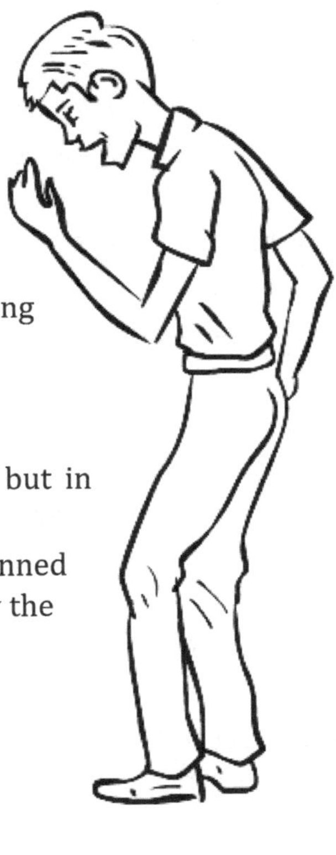

- A cough that lasts longer than 3 weeks, often worse just after waking up.
- Slight fever in the evening and sweating at night.
- There may be pain in the chest or upper back.
- Chronic loss of weight and increasing weakness.

In serious or advanced cases:

- Coughing up blood (usually a little, but in some cases a lot).
- Pale, waxy skin. The skin of a dark skinned person tends to get lighter, especially the face.
- Voice grows hoarse (very serious).

In young children:

- Steady weight loss.
- Frequent fever.
- Lighter skin color.
- Swelling in the neck (lymph nodes) or in the belly.

Cure:

- Mix gooseberry juice with honey and take that on a daily basis.
- Consume bottle gourd (lauki) juice .

Juice Therapy:

- Drink 200 ml of apple juice daily.
- Drink grape juice.
- Drink carrot juice.

ANEMIA

Symptoms

- Blood is lost or destroyed faster than the body can replace it.
- Pale or transparent skin.
- Pale inside of eyelids.
- White fingernails.
- Pale gums.
- Weakness and fatigue.

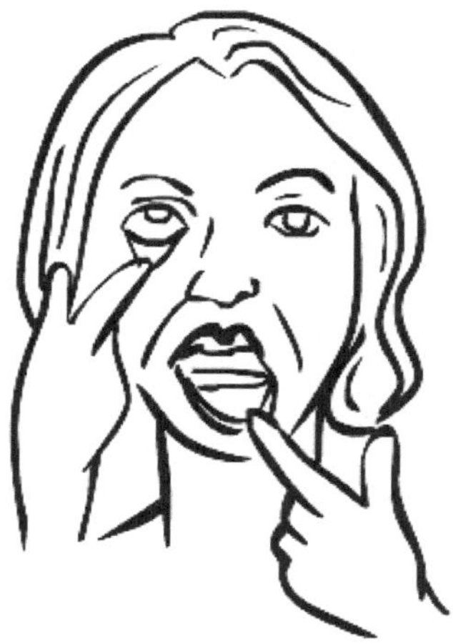

Cure:

- Take 50 ml of wheatgrass juice twice a day preferably on an empty stomach.

Juice Therapy:

- Drink strawberries, broccoli and citrus juice.
- Extract juice of one half cup fresh spinach, two celery stalks, three carrots, one half lemon and one half beet and drink on a daily basis.

HIGH BLOOD PRESSURE (HYPERTENSION)

Symptoms

- Frequent headaches.
- Pounding of the heart and shortness of breath with mild exercise.

- Weakness and dizziness.
- Occasional pain in the left shoulder and chest.

Cure:

- Eat 1 or 2 crushed garlic cloves daily.
- Mix1 tsp honey with 1 tsp ginger and 1 tsp cumin powder and have it twice a day.

Juice therapy:

- Drink celery juice.
- Drink watermelon juice.

CONSTIPATION

Symptoms

- Hard stool.
- No bowel movement for 3 or more days.

Cure:

- Drink hot water with 1 tsp honey and juice of 1/2 lemon first thing in the morning.
- Drink water which has been kept overnight in a copper vessel first thing in the morning.
- Drink 1 liter water in the morning in one go.
- Drink aloe vera juice.

Juice Therapy:

- Drink juice of dark green leafy vegetables.
- Drink pumpkin juice.
- Drink raw cucumber juice.
- Start the day with the blend of equal parts of apple, beet root and carrot along with 1 tsp ginger juice.

DIABETES

- Always thirsty.
- Urinates (pees) often and a lot.
- Always tired.
- Always hungry.
- Weight loss.
- Itchy skin.
- Periods of blurry eyesight.
- Some loss of feeling in hands or feet.
- Frequent vaginal infections.
- Sores on the feet that do not heal.
- Loss of consciousness (in extreme cases).

Cure:

- Chew 10 - 15 basil leaves in the morning.
- Take 1 tbs of amla juice mixed with honey daily.
- Drink a glass of lukewarm water with freshly squeezed lemon juice.
- Consume 10-30 ml of Aloe-Vera juice daily on an empty stomach in the morning.

Juice Therapy:

- Consume 1 tbs of amla juice mixed with a cup of bitter gourd juice daily for two months.
- Drink french beans juice.
- Drink pear juice.

ACID INDIGESTION, HEARTBURN, AND STOMACH ULCERS

Symptoms

- Discomfort or a burning feeling in the stomach or mid chest.
- Pain gets worse when lying down.

- Vomiting with fresh blood or with digested blood stools with blood.

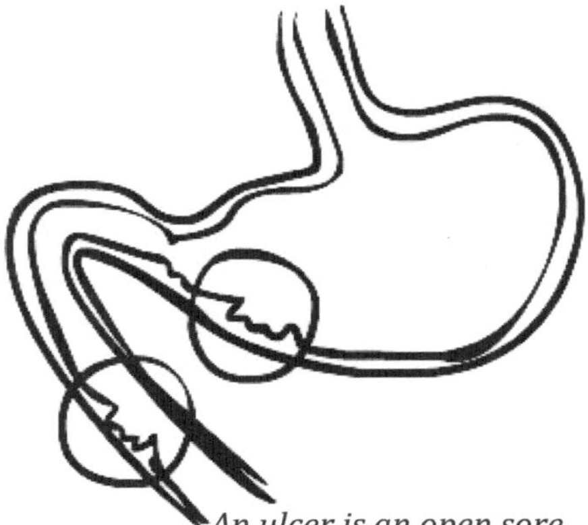

An ulcer is an open sore in the stomach or gut.

Cure:

- Drink two glasses of water in the morning.
- Consume tulsi leaves on regular basis.
- Chew a small piece of ginger with salt 5 to 10 minutes before meal.
- Consume 10 ml to 20 ml aloe vera juice two - three times a day.

Juice Therapy:

- Drink spinach juice.
- Drink 200 ml of broccoli and spinach juice daily.
- Drink a cup of potato juice.

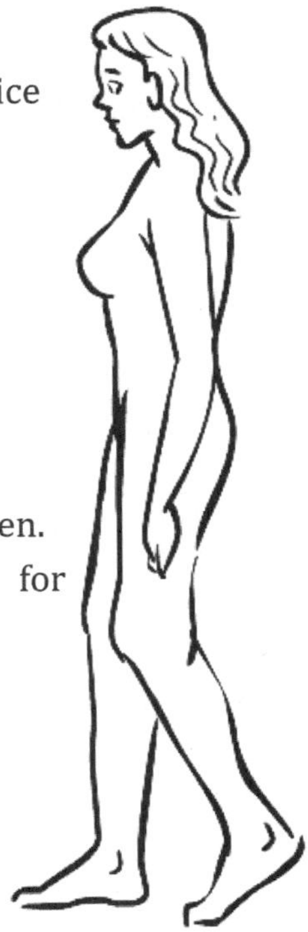

URINARY TRACT INFECTIONS

- Fever and chills or headache.
- Pain in the side.
- Painful urination and urge to urinate very often.
- Unable to hold in urine (especially true for children).
- Urine may be cloudy or reddish (bloody).
- Pain in the lower back (kidneys).
- Feet and face may swell.

Cure:

- Drink plenty of water.
- Drink cranberry juice.
- Urinate frequently.
- Avoid coffee, alcohol, and soft drinks containing citrus juices or caffeine.

BLADDER STONE

Symptoms

- Sharp or severe pain in the lower back & lower belly.
- Difficulty in passing urine.
- Drops of blood while urinating.
- Urinary infection

Cure:

- Consume basil juice mixed with honey for 6 months.
- Add 2 tsp finely grounded coriander seeds in a glass of boiling hot water. Add honey to taste.

Juice Therapy:

- Drink coconut water.
- Drink banana pulp juice.
- Drink watermelon juice.
- Consume lemon juice.
- Drink grape juice.

ENLARGED PROSTATE GLAND

Symptoms

- Difficulty in passing urine and bowel movement.
- Urine may dribble or drip or become blocked completely.

- Not able to urinate for days.
- Fever

Cure:

- If the person cannot urinate, try sitting in a tub of hot water as shown in the picture.
- Consume pumpkin seeds.
- Drink 8 glasses of water a day.
- Limit your intake of fatty foods.

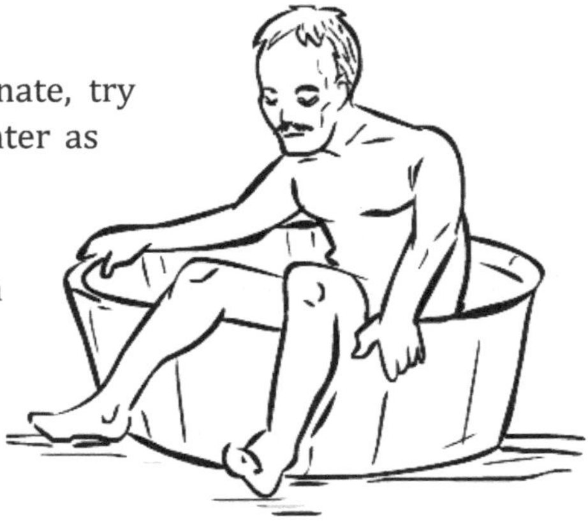

VAGINAL DISCHARGE

Symptoms

- A mucus or pus like stuff that comes from the vagina.
- A thin and foamy, greenish yellow or whitish, foul smelling discharge with itching.
- White discharge that looks like cottage cheese or buttermilk, and smells like mold, mildew or baking bread.
- Thick, milky discharge with a rancid smell.
- Watery, brown or gray discharge, streaked with blood, bad smell, pain in lower belly.

Cure:

- Mix the juice of basil leaves and honey in equal proportion and take it in the morning and evening for two weeks.
- Eat one to two overripe bananas daily to help control vaginal discharge.
- Drink cranberry juice three times a day.

PAIN OR DISCOMFORT IN A WOMAN'S BELLY

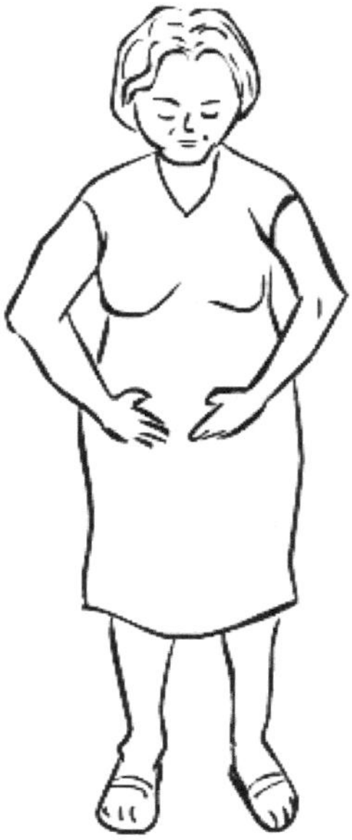

- Menstrual discomfort.
- A bladder infection.
- Pelvic inflammatory disease.
- Lump or mass in the lower part of the belly.
- Ectopic pregnancy.
- Infection or other problem of the gut or rectum.

Cure:

- Fomentation or Hot Sitz Bath.
- Mix 2 teaspoons of lime juice in 50 ml of warm water and add honey to it. Drink it at least thrice a day.

PAINFUL MENSTRUAL PERIOD

Do's

- Walk around.
- Do light work.
- Do light exercises.
- Take hot drinks.
- Soak feet in hot water.

Don'ts

- Do-not lie down or stay in bed.

EMERGENCY DELIVERIES (CHILD BIRTH)

Types of Emergency Deliveries:

1. Labor Stops or Slows Down
2. Breech Delivery

3. Cord Wrapped around the Baby's Neck
4. Feces in the Baby's Mouth and Nose

1. Labor Stops or Slows Down

Causes:

i) The woman may be frightened or upset:

Cure:

- Talk to the woman, relax her.
- Drink Plenty of Water.
- Drink Fruit Juices.
- Eat lots of Fruits and Vegetables.
- Urinate frequently.
- Massage of the nipples.

ii) If the baby is facing forward:

Cure:

- Woman should change position often.
- Have her try on her hands and knees to turn the baby.

iii) If the mother has been vomiting too much:

Cure:

- Drink lot of water
- Drink coconut water frequently.
- Drink fruit juices.

2. Breech Delivery

Case 1:

If the baby's legs come out first

Steps:

1. Wash your hands with alcohol or wear gloves.

2. Slip your fingers inside and push the baby's shoulders toward the back.
3. or press his arms against his body.
4. Put your finger in the baby's mouth and push his head towards his chest.
5. Have someone push the baby's head down by pressing on the mother's belly.
6. Have the mother push hard.
7. Do not pull on the body of the baby.

3. Cord is Wrapped Around the Baby's Neck

Steps:

1. Slip the loop of cord from around the baby's neck.
2. Clamp or tie and cut the cord using blunt tipped scissors.

4. Feces in the Baby's Mouth snd Nose

Symptoms:

When the water break, if you see they contain a dark green liquid.

Steps:

1. As soon as head is out, tell the mother not to push.
2. Suck the feces out of baby's nose and mouth with suction pump.
3. Keeping sucking until you get all the feces out.

Note:

Note:

SECTION

V

This section is devoted to two of the illness i.e. Cancer and Mental Disorders which among all the diseases are at forefront and responsible for reducing the quality of life and also the shortening of the life span. It is a well known fact that 20% of the modern men die of cancer and every 4th person suffers from some kind of mental illness in his life time. This section will teach you methods to relieve the mankind from the two main causes of human suffering.

CANCER

What is Cancer?

Understanding Cancer will be easy if you understand the fact "Why there is no heart cancer?" You will note further in this section that there is brain cancer, breast cancer, lung cancer, colon cancer but there is no heart cancer.

Simple steps of cancer formation:

Step 1: Blockage is formed in a particular location of the blood vessel leading to the deprivation of food & oxygen to the nearby cells.

Step 2: In the absence of food & oxygen the cells have no choice but to die especially if it is the cells of heart. This leads to heart disease.

Step 3: Except heart cells, cells of other organs of the body may decide not to die, but to steal food & oxygen from the nearby organ, where the supply of blood is still abundant.

Step 4: The cells (deprived of food & oxygen) make micro blood vessels to steal food & oxygen from nearby vessels. This process is called angiogenesis.

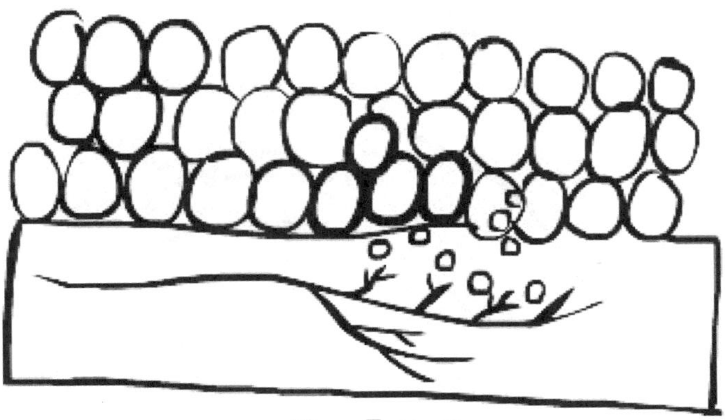

Micro Tumour

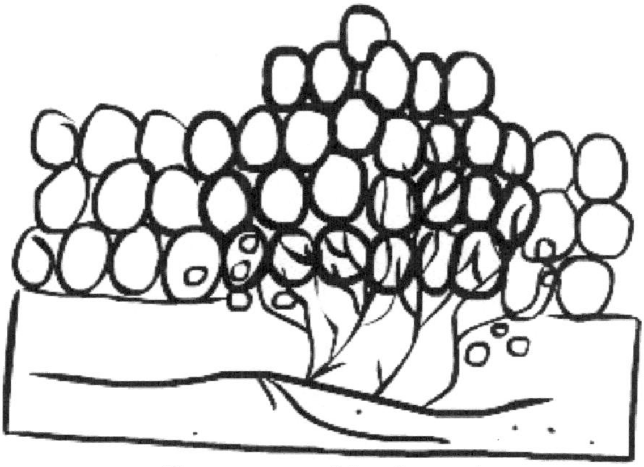

Tumour capable of growing and invading other tissues

ANGIOGENESIS

Step 5: This uncontrolled stolen supply of food & oxygen to otherwise starved cells leads to uncontrolled growth and multiplication of cells called as tumor.

Step 6: These primary tumor cells most often migrate to other part of the body, transported by the blood, which results in spreading of cancer to different organs also called as metastasis.

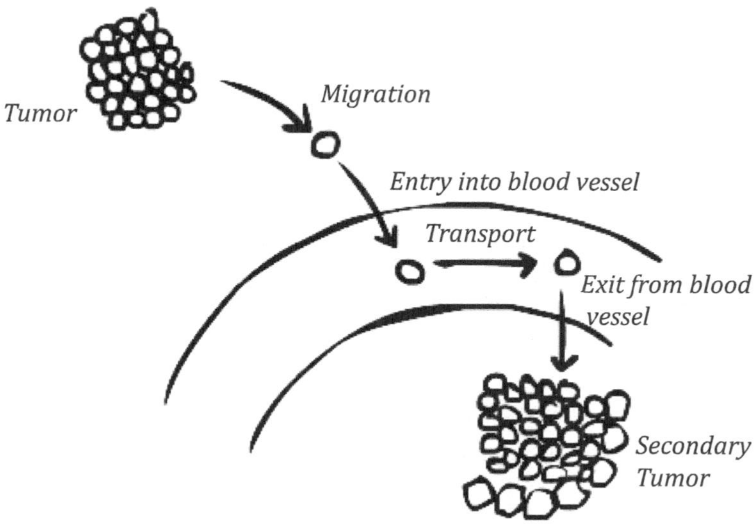

STEPS OF METASTASIS

More than 90% of the cancer deaths are due to Metastasis.

Types of Cancer:

BLADDER CANCER

Symptoms

- Blood in the urine, turning in red or rusty – colored.
- Feeling a need to urinate but nothing comes out.
- Painful or urgent urination.

BREAST CANCER

Symptoms:

In women:

- Lump or mass in the breast found by breast exam.
- Firm or hard; irregular borders; usually painless.
- Change in size or shape of one breast.
- Change in color or feel of the skin of the breast, areola (pigmented skin around the nipple), or nipple of one breast.
- Puckered or scaly.
- Redness
- Enlargement, itching, or retraction (pulling in) of nipple.
- (Advanced disease) Bone pain, swelling in one arm, weight loss, ulceration of the skin of the breast.

In men:

- Any breast lump & pain, or tenderness.

COLORECTAL CANCER

Symptoms

- Constipation or diarrhea lasting 2 weeks or more.
- Darker stools.
- Dark (not bright red) blood in (not on) the stool, or bright red

blood (not dark) on (not in) the stool.

- Anemia that cannot be otherwise explained.

LIVER CANCER

Symptoms

- Bloating, abdominal swelling may be severe.
- Fever
- Loss of appetite.
- Pain in the upper abdomen on the right side; the pain may extend to the back and shoulder.
- Weakness or severe fatigue.
- Weight loss.
- Yellow skin and eyes, and dark urine (jaundice).
- Liver cancer may present no symptoms in its early stages.

LUNG CANCER

Symptoms

- New onset of persistent cough, especially if you smoke.
- Shortness of breath.
- Dull chest pain (does not always occur).
- Coughing up blood (It does not always occur).

OVARIAN CANCER

Symptoms

- Abdominal swelling.
- Lumps or masses in the abdomen.
- Vaginal bleeding.
- Difficult urination.
- Lower back pain.

PANCREATIC CANCER

Symptoms

The outward symptoms of pancreatic cancer are especially vague and are associated with many other diseases. Most patients with treatable pancreatic cancer have very few symptoms.

Having any or all of these symptoms should not be interpreted as evidence of pancreatic cancer.

- Blood in stool.
- Dark urine and light stools.
- Loss of appetite.
- Pain over the stomach that is worse after eating.
- Weight loss.
- Yellowing of the skin.

PROSTATE CANCER

Symptoms

- Difficulty in starting or stopping stream of urine.
- Increased frequency of urination.
- Pain while urinating.
- Blood in urine (rare).
- Importance (rare as a result of the disease itself).

BASAL CELL CARCINOMA

Symptoms

- A pink growth with a slightly elevated center, from which tiny blood vessel may be radiating, or
- A shiny bump or nodule that is translucent pink, red or white, or
- An open sore that bleeds, oozes, or crusts and remains open for 3 or more weeks, or
- Reddened skin or irritation on the arms, chest, face, or legs that persists for 3 or more weeks, with or without itching, or

- A waxy, white, or yellow scar like area, sometimes with a crust (This is a sign of an especially aggressive variety of this form of cancer).
- In all forms of basal cell carcinoma, very mild trauma, such as washing or drying with a towel, may cause bleeding.
- Basal cell carcinomas are less common on black or dark skin, but will usually contain concentrated black or brown pigment.

How to cure cancer:

By now you might have clearly understood that although there are different kinds of symptoms and effects of cancer on the patients but the basic mechanism by which the cancer cell is formed is same i.e. angiogenesis. Even in the case of the blood cancer, angiogenesis takes place in bone marrow.

Since the basic cause of all cancer is the same i.e. the formation of angiogenic blood vessels for the uncontrolled supply of food & oxygen to the otherwise food deficient cells. An anti angiogenesis approach for cure can help a patient recover from the disease.

This means blocking the angiogenic blood vessels leading to cancer cells starve to death.

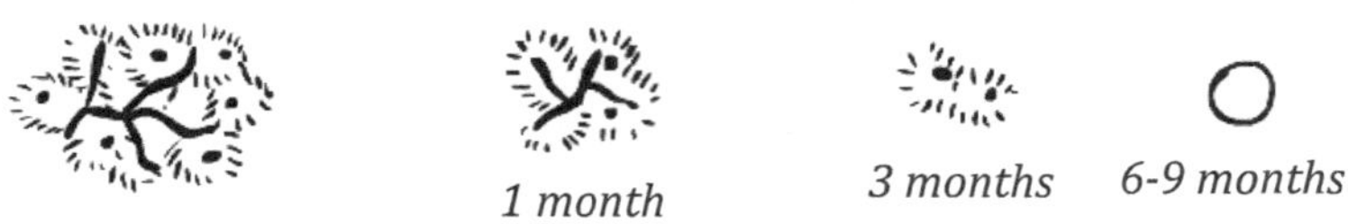

How to block the food & oxygen supply to cancer cells:

According to the noble prize winning science - 1998, body produces a miracle molecule called Nitric Oxide (NO), which if produced in abundance can block the angiogenic blood vessels leading to the death of cancer cells. Certain kind of food (Cancer Diet) can help the body to produce Nitric Oxide in abundance leading to the recovery from cancer.

FLOW CHART FOR CANCER RECOVERY

Cancer Diet for 6 -9 months

↓

Body ability to produce Nitric Oxide is enhanced

↓

All angiogenic blood vessels are blocked

↓

Food & Oxygen supply to cancer cells stops

↓

Recovery from cancer

The Cancer Diet:

To recover from cancer the patient must follow the diet based on the table given below:

1	Milk & dairy products	0%
2	Animal food	0%
3	Salt, sugar & oil	0%
4	Packed & refined food	0%
5	Raw green leaves & vegetables	25%
6	Other raw vegetables	25%
7	Sprouts	5%
8	Grains	10%
9	Nuts	5%
10	Fruits	30%
11	Cooked Foods	Negligible
12	Sunlight exposure	At least 1 hr everyday

Eating food based on the above table for 6 to 9 months can help a patient to recover from Cancer.

MENTAL ILLNESS

What is Mental Illness?

Unlike other animals of the planet, man is a social animal, bound by certain rules, regulations and also by expectations about the way he must behave and lead his life in relation to rest of the society. Any deviation from the expected behavior may be labelled as a mental illness.

The present understanding of the mental illness is being classified in 5 major categories:

1. Disorders diagnosed in childhood : ADHD, ADD
2. Cognitive Disorder: Mental illness as a result of life style disease.
3. Substance related disease: Alcohol, caffeine.
4. Mood disorder: Depression
5. Situation related disorder: Phobia, anxiety.

Causes of Mental Illness:

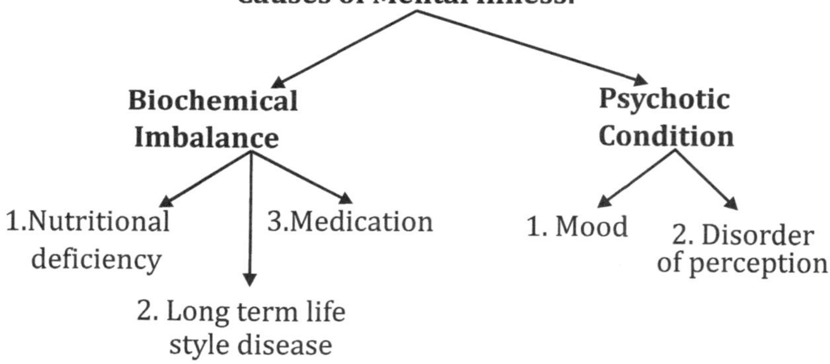

Most of the time, the mental illness is because of the combination of both the above causes.

The indicators of the biochemical imbalance of the brain:

You may ask the patient the following statements:

- People's faces sometimes pulsate as I watch them.
- People watch me all the time.
- Now and then when I look in the mirror my face changes and it seems different.

- Sometimes when I read, the words begin to look funny - they move around or grow faint.
- Sometimes objects pulsate when I look at them.
- My hands or feet sometimes seem much too large for me.
- I sometimes feel that I have left my body.
- I often hear or have heard voices.
- I can no longer tell how much time has gone by.
- I often hear thoughts inside my head.
- I find that past, present and future all seem muddled up.

The presence of symptoms such as these suggests that something isn't right in the way the brain is processing information, which is a good indicator that a person has biochemical imbalance.

This means treatment of such patients should be more focused towards recommending the patient a special diet for mental illness to recover the brain function.

However we must understand that one cause leads to the other.

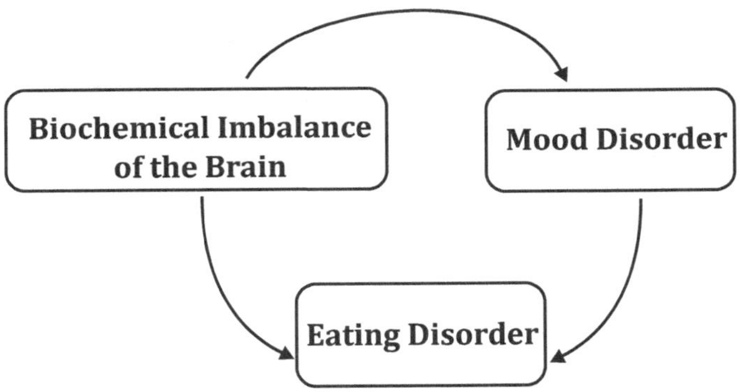

And also there is a trouble in the diagnosis and the categorization of the disease in mental illness patients because of the two main reasons:

Reason 1: There is a great amount of similarity in symptoms of various types of mental illnesses.

Reason 2: The patients' symptoms keep on changing on a continuous basis. With the change in the symptoms patients switch from one mental illness to the other. For example, a Schizophrenia patient may be diagnosed as a patient of bipolar disease and after some time he may be showing the symptoms of a patient with severe depression.

Given below are the symptoms of some common mental illnesses. You can easily notice the similarity of symptoms among various mental illnesses.

ADD/ADHD

(Attention Deficit Disorder / Attention Deficit Hyperactivity Disorder) in Children

Symptoms:

Attention Deficit:

- Difficulty in maintaining attention to work or play.
- Easily distracted.
- Failure to pay attention to details & makes careless mistakes at school or work.
- Has difficulty in organizing tasks or time.
- Unable to follow instructions unless they are given one at a time.

HYPERACTIVITY:

- Runs or climbs in inappropriate situations.
- Thumping, fidgeting, squirming, moving constantly.

Associated Symptoms:

- Learning disabilities.
- Social isolation, although may relate well one-on-one.

ALZHEIMER'S DISEASE

Symptoms:

Early Stages:

- Getting lost on familiar routes.

- Losing interest in activities once enjoyed.
- Misplacing familiar objects.
- Personality changes.
- Repeating statements frequently.
- Trouble finding names for familiar objects.

More advanced Stages:

- Decreased knowledge of recent events.
- Delusions, depression, and agitation.
- Forgetting events in personal history.
- Hallucinations, arguments, striking out, and violent behavior.
- Problems choosing proper clothing.

BIPOLAR DISORDER

(Manic Depression)

Symptoms:

- Bipolar disorder causes alternating periods of depression, mania and possibly psychosis.

Depression:

A depressive episode is diagnosed if 5 or more of the following symptoms last most of the day, nearly every day, for a period of 2 weeks or longer.

- Change in appetite and/or unintended weight loss or gain.
- Difficulty in concentrating and making decisions, as well as memory loss.
- Feelings of guilt, helplessness, hopelessness, or worthlessness.
- Lasting anxious, empty, or sad mood.
- Loss of interest in activities once enjoyed including sex.
- Restlessness or irritability.
- Sleeping too much or inability to sleep.
- Thoughts of death or suicide or suicide attempts.

MANIA

- A period of behavior that is different from usual, lasting up to 1 week.
- Abuse of drugs, particularly cocaine, alcohol, and sleeping medications.
- Denial that anything is wrong.
- Excessively "high", overly good mood.
- Extreme irritability
- Inability to concentrate
- Poor judgment
- Provocative, intrusive or aggressive behavior.

Psychosis:

- Delusion (false, strongly held beliefs not influenced by logical reasoning or explained by a person's usual cultural concepts).
- Hallucinations in hearing, seeing, or otherwise sensing the presence of things not actually there)

EPILEPSY

Symptoms:

Seizures:

- Tonic (stiffening of the body, dilation of the pupils).
- Clonic (sudden muscle jerks)
- Atonic (loss of muscle tone and/or consciousness).

Obsessive-Compulsive Disorder (OCD)

Symptoms:

- Persistent or recurrent ideas or impulses that cause distress.
- International purposeful and repetitive behaviors performed in response to an obsession.

PARKINSON'S DISEASE

Symptoms:

- Tremors at rest.
- Rigidity
- Slow initiation of movement.
- Two out of 3 symptoms is required to make a diagnosis of the disease.
- Postural instability, difficulty remaining upright, occurs after 8 or more years the disease begins.

Other possible symptoms include:

- Altered vision.
- Altered mental status.
- Flexed posture of arms and neck.

SCHIZOPHRENIA

Symptoms:

- Delusions (beliefs held despite evidence to the contrary).
- Hallucinations (usually hearing, sometimes seeing, things that do not physically exist).
- Loss of appetite.
- Social withdrawl.
- Loss of Hygiene.
- Sense of being controlled from the outside.

TENSION HEADACHES

Symptoms:

- Dull pain and pressure on both sides of the head.
- No sense of pulsation.
- Sensitivity to light or sound but not both.
- May last from 30 minutes to a week.
- No nausea or vomiting.
- Not aggravated by physical activity.

- Not associated with a prodrome in which "you can feel it coming on".

Diet for mentally ill patient to recover from the biochemical imbalance of the brain:

1	Animal food including milk products	0%
2	All refined & packed foods	0%
3	Citrus fruits	25%
4	Other fruits	7-8%
5	Nuts	35%
6	Grains	25%
7	Raw Vegetables	5%
8	Sunshine	More than 30 minutes
9	Physical exercise	About 1/2 hrs

Total Time to recover: - Nearly one Year

Strategy to recover from the psychotic condition and Mood Disorder

The patient must read the following rules everyday and try to implement the rules given in his/her life.

1. According to research, worrying makes you tense and nervous and affects the nerves of your stomach. It actually changes the gastric juices of your stomach and often leads to stomach ulcers.

"Those who do not know how to fight worry, die young."

- Dr. Alexis Carrel

2. One of the worst features of 'worry' is that it destroys our ability to concentrate. When we worry, our mind runs haywire and we lose all the power of decision. However, when we force ourselves to face the worst and accept it mentally, then we

eliminate all these vague imaginations and put ourselves in a position where we are able to concentrate on our problems.

3. **Do this**: Analyze the situation fearlessly and honestly and figure out the worst that could happen as a result of the failure. After that, calmly devote your time and energy to improve upon the worst which you have already accepted mentally.

4 Carefully read the sentence given below:

A man is not hurt so much by what happened, as by his opinion of 'what happened'. Now follow this unique technique to change your opinion and mood instantly. Action seems to follow feeling, but actually action and feeling go hand in hand and by regulating the action which is under the direct control of our will, we can indirectly regulate the feeling, which is not under our control.

So, act as if you are happy; speak and walk cheerfully as if you are already cheerful and if possible, even dance for a moment.

Remember the words of Abraham Lincoln;

"Most folks are about as happy they make up their mind to be."

5. I had blues because I had no shoes, until upon the street; I met a man who had no feet.

Read this every morning and you will never have worries for the things you do not have.

6 **Visualization Technique**: Keep a mental account of the happier moments of your life. Next time you are tense, go back to your happier days by visualizing yourself in that moment. Try to feel the pleasant atmosphere and music of appreciation of your happier moment.

"We are not what we are, but what we think we are."

Note:

Note: